Well-Being
and Well-Dying,
Cancel the Cancer

Well-Being
and Well-Dying,
Cancel the Cancer

Min Young Lee

SFJ Pharmaceuticals Group, Singapore

World Scientific

NEW JERSEY · LONDON · SINGAPORE · BEIJING · SHANGHAI · HONG KONG · TAIPEI · CHENNAI · TOKYO

Published by

World Scientific Publishing Co. Pte. Ltd.

5 Toh Tuck Link, Singapore 596224

USA office: 27 Warren Street, Suite 401-402, Hackensack, NJ 07601

UK office: 57 Shelton Street, Covent Garden, London WC2H 9HE

Library of Congress Cataloging-in-Publication Data

Names: Lee, Min (Min Young), author.

Title: Well-being and well-dying : cancel the cancer / Min Young Lee.

Description: New Jersey : World Scientific, [2018] | Includes bibliographical references.

Identifiers: LCCN 2018037038| ISBN 9789813273191 (hardcover : alk. paper) |
    ISBN 9813273194 (hardcover : alk. paper)

Subjects: LCSH: Cancer--Patients. | Cancer--Treatment.

Classification: LCC RC263 .L366 2018 | DDC 616.99/4--dc23

LC record available at https://lccn.loc.gov/2018037038

British Library Cataloguing-in-Publication Data

A catalogue record for this book is available from the British Library.

First published 2019 (Hardcover)

Reprinted 2019 (in paperback edition)

ISBN 978-981-3275-08-9 (pbk)

For any available supplementary material, please visit
https://www.worldscientific.com/worldscibooks/10.1142/11068#t=suppl

Well-Being and Well-Dying, Cancel the Cancer

Prologue

During a BIO US conference held in Boston several years ago, there was a reception organized by Harvard University. Many scientists and businessmen were invited to the reception, and they gathered around to listen to the opening speech offered by the Director of Business Development at Harvard University. The question and answer that was exchanged during his speech still lingers in my memory today.

The question was: "Harvard University is one of the best university in the world, in which many prestigious professors are teaching students and conducting research in area of science and technology. These professors have been working and leading scientific research in many ways, and they have built up tremendous academic achievements. They have been carrying out research with tremendous amount of research fund over the past few decades. Now, where are the results of the research that have been funded for decades?"

Everyone tuned their ears to hear the answer from the speaker. After a few seconds of pause, he said, "Well, most of the research results went into the bookshelves of University Library." As you might have already understood the intention of this question and answer, the message he wanted to deliver was that research results should be something substantial that can bring realistic benefits for human being. The substantial benefits may include new technologies or products developed that are useful for consumers.

Consumers are purchasing and using various types of products provided from various industries. Consumers can purchase most household products by themselves for use. However, consumers cannot buy specialty products such as medicines and medical devices by themselves, and these medical or pharmaceutical products should be purchased and used via the prescription of medical doctors or pharmacists. As laymen consumers may have limited scientific or medical knowledge about the specialty products that could be accompanied with side effects or unexpected risk, they will need to rely on licensed experts or medical doctors to purchase the medical or pharmaceutical products.

Consumers may regress to a state of naivety when they get struck with a disease, due to limited knowledge about the disease. They may become vulnerable to various different opinions or comments on a variety of treatment options for their disease, making them even more confused. However, if the information about the disease and the medical treatment options are easily communicated and understood by the end users, i.e., patients, then patients themselves will be able to react more positively to the disease and achieve a better quality of life, with the help and medical support from the hospital.

The author is a Scientist who studied in Life Sciences. More specifically, he graduated with Ph.D. in Toxicology from Oregon State University and worked as a researcher at the Institute of Chemical Toxicology in Wayne State University. After that, he worked for US FDA. After FDA, he joined Procter and Gamble US and worked for many years in the area of Regulatory and

Human Safety. After P&G, he worked on the clinical development of pharmaceutical drugs as CEO of CMIC Korea. After CMIC, he led Business Development, Research & Development of new drugs, and the Commercialization of biosimilar drugs at Korean conglomerate companies. He had been an Adjunct Professor in Department of Life Science of Korea University for six years (2008–2013). Currently, he is President of Asia Pacific, SFJ Pharmaceuticals Group, responsible for clinical operations of new cancer drug development in the Asia Pacific region.

The author believes that the knowledge and experiences learned from the industry should not be confined to the industry itself, but be made practically useful for the ordinary consumers, via easy communication and interpretation of the knowledge. With this philosophy, the author wrote this book in attempt to help ordinary people understand the cancer disease and its medical science, with easy-to-understand wordings, so that patients can manage cancer more effectively in their lifetime.

Acknowledgments

I would like to acknowledge the citing of wonderful information and data available from public internet sites, as well as many cancer-related research articles published and announced by leading cancer research organizations, such as National Cancer Institute (NCI), American Society of Clinical Oncology (ASCO), and American Association for Cancer Research (AACR), etc. In addition, I humbly acknowledge the rewording or copying of some wordings written by unidentified people in the Internet space, who should deserve to get some credits.

With this opportunity, I would like to send my sincere gratitude to many people, who had helped me in my career progression, as my advisors or mentors through the past decades. Firstly, thanks to Dr. George S. Bailey and Dr. David E. Williams in Oregon State University, who admitted me to the doctorate toxicology program with a research assistantship. Secondly, thanks to Dr. Ronald W. Hart, Ex-Director of NCTR/ US FDA, who provided me with the opportunity to work on National Toxicology Program. Thirdly, thanks to CEO Naka- mura, founder of CMIC Japan, providing me an opportunity to lead the CRO business. Fourthly, thanks to my esteemed friend, Robert Debenedetto, founder and CEO of SFJ Phar- maceuticals Group, providing me the opportunity to operate global clinical studies with oncology drugs.

I also would like to thank my fellow colleague, Faith Fung, for sharing her experience in fighting breast cancer, as well as helping to edit the manuscript. In addition, the team from the publisher, World Scientific, for finishing the book with detailed editing of the contents.

Finally, I would like to send my deep love and appreciation to my mother P. B. Choi and father ex-H. D. Lee, who devoted their whole life to the success and prosperity of their children.

Reviewers' Comments

REVIEWER 1

David Read, MPH
Vice President of Medical Oncology
Dana-Farber Cancer Institute*
450 Brookline Ave. Suite 1608
Boston, MA 02215

Well-Being and Well-Dying, Cancel the Cancer provides a broad overview of where we are in the early 21st century regarding

---

*A principal teaching affiliate of Harvard Medical School.

the battle to understand and treat this long standing scurge on humanity. The book balances the right tone, length and level of complexity for patients, families, and lay persons, who are seeking to understand this disease for themselves, friends or loved-ones. The author references some of the more recent academic journal articles by leading experts who are having a significant impact in the understanding and treatment of cancer.

The book starts with a clear and articulate overview of cancer biology at the cellular and organ system level. Next, the author delves into the principles of the toxicology and drug concepts used to treat cancer. The book contains excellent illustrations and graphical displays of the issues related to cancers. It was refreshing to read how much of an overview of basic science, translational and clinical research has been summarized in this important work for patients and families — and the public in general. The author references the most up to date research that is currently available. This book also provides an excellent explanation of the stages and grades of cancer for patients, families and the public.

As importantly, this work also addresses the understandable anxiety that patients feel with a new or recurring cancer diagnosis. In the world of oncology, there is an increased awareness to help and take care of the whole patient — not just treat their tumors. As all cancers can't be cured, yet, the book provides a good segway to palliative medicine, hospice care and unfortunately for some — death and dying. It provides both a realistic view of the cancer and the broad spectrum of outcomes, what is currently being done to combat the disease, and also hope for the future.

In summary, I would highly recommend this book to any patients who has recently been diagnosed with cancer. With some further editing for an American audience, this body of work will be a valuable resource. I am very much looking forward to recommending this book to our patient and family resource center and helping make it available this work in the book section of our gift shop at Dana-Farber Cancer Institute.

REVIEWER 2

Robert DeBenedetto
President and CEO, SFJ Pharmaceuticals, Inc.
5000 Hopyard Road, Suite #330
Pleasanton, CA 94566

There are many books that describe what cancer is, and other books that describe the various types of drug treatment; however, this book *Well-Being and Well-Dying, Cancel the Cancer* encapsulates not only a description of what cancer is, and how to treat it, but in addition in layman terms the book explains, what is the root cause of many cancers and probably more importantly, how to live a life to reduce your chances of getting cancer in the first place.

The author's having lived and worked in the United States, Japan and Singapore, in addition to his home country of South Korea, has provided him the unique exposure to lifestyles of cancer patients and the cancer treatment regimens used in various regions of the world. The author's global experience has also exposed him to the fact, that it does not matter in which country a person may live, the news that they are diagnosed with cancer creates the same emotional reactions and progression of feelings as a patient goes from hearing the initial news of their disease, through disbelief, anger, acceptance, etc. as the patient goes through their various treatment options to either the success of conquering and surviving cancer or to the arrival of final end-of-life decisions.

There are painful truths that are hard to put in writing, but are necessary to be said for the cancer patient's complete understanding and reflection, which I applaud the author for his courage to say the words that many people prefer not to hear, but need to hear.

This book is a virtual encyclopedia that provides answers to almost any question a cancer patient will ultimately need to ask, from what causes cancer in the first place, what types and stages of cancer are there, what are the treatment options, the pros and cons of entering a clinical trial, the right time to seek hospice care, and end-of-life decision that a patient in some cases will need to make.

As the President and CEO of a pharmaceutical company that develops new cancer fighting drugs, our trials touch thousands of cancer patient lives every day. Based on this experience, I strongly recommend this book as a must read for cancer patients in all stages of their disease.

REVIEWER 3

Rolf Linke, MD
Physician and Clinical Researcher
Chief Medical Officer, SFJ Pharmaceuticals
Duernberg 6
D-83417 Kirchanschoering
Germany

Dr. Lee did a fantastic job in describing important and complex aspects of cancer in a very interesting and generally under-standable way and shares helpful considerations for people dealing with cancer or people caring for cancer patients. With his background and experiences in toxicology and clinical development, he summarizes major risk factors for development of cancer and describes strategies to minimize them; explains relevant aspects of cancer which a patient may face, including diagnostics and characterization of tumors, treatment and care options without going deep into technical details. This is a well written compendium which could be very helpful for professional staff dealing with cancer patients but also for lay person facing this malignant disease.

REVIEWER 4

Faith Fung, Ph.D., MBA
Vice President, Clinical Development, Asia
SFJ Pharmaceuticals Asia Pacific Pte. Ltd.
41 Science Park Road, #04-02 The Gemini, Singapore 117610.
And a Breast Cancer Survivor

Shock, fear, confusion and denial are common feelings that overtake our emotions when one is first diagnosed with cancer. Next, it will be followed by a flurry of activities arranged by the hospital staff for surgery, chemotherapy, radiotherapy, pain management, physiotherapy, alternative therapy, etc. So for the patient, the next six months or longer will be spent going from one clinic appointment to another, just like a mouse on a running wheel, incessant running around with no end in sight.

For most patients, the "cancer" diagnosis is like a cruel death sentence to a seemingly happy life. Upon diagnosis, most are taken aback or frozen into inaction. There is a vacuum of not knowing what to do next. Many patients may not have much knowledge about cancer and treatment options, and would be anxious to know what can be done. Family members or friends may also offer a variety of advice that may further confuse the patient.

In actual fact, cancer research and cancer therapy have advanced significantly in the past decade. A cancer diagnosis no longer needs to equate to a death sentence. Many new, personalized, targeted cancer therapy have been found to significantly prolong survival, even in late stage cancer patients. In addition, these new cancer drugs also come with much less side effects, compared to conventional chemotherapy. Hence, cancer patients can still live on for a long period of time, after diagnosis.

The author wrote this book to help people understand the cancer disease and its medical science, so patients can manage cancer more effectively in their lifetime. Providing information for patients to understand their treatment plan can help reduce anxiety and give them a greater sense of ownership. This sense of ownership is imperative to growing a positive attitude for patients fighting cancer.

This book is a MUST for cancer patients, family members of cancer patients, supportive care staff, medical students, pharmacy students and staff, science students and anyone interested in knowing more about cancer. This book is a very good cancer reference book for the current generation and future generations.

Diagrams Showing How People are Exposed to Toxic Chemical Substances and How Cancer Cells are Formed After Gene Mutations Occur through Active Toxic Chemical Compounds

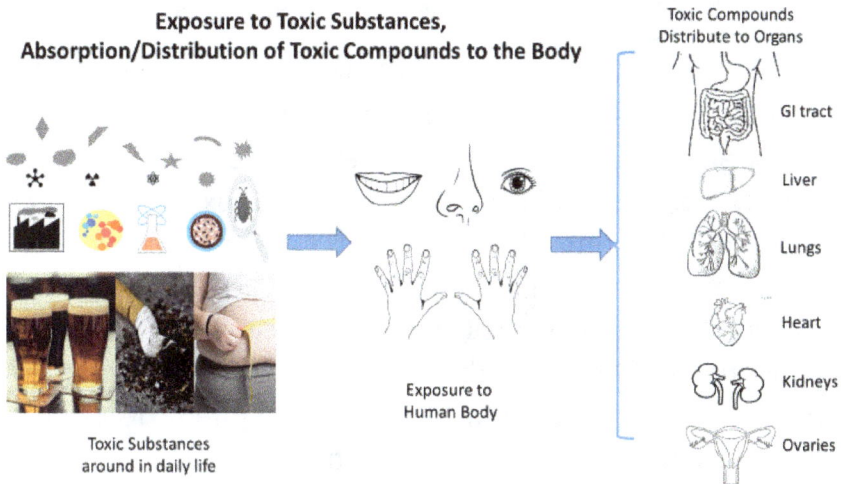

Exposure to Toxic Substances, Absorption/Distribution of Toxic Compounds to the Body

Toxic Substances around in daily life

Exposure to Human Body

Toxic Compounds Distribute to Organs

GI tract

Liver

Lungs

Heart

Kidneys

Ovaries

People are exposed to chemical substances from the environment and the use of household goods every day. These chemical substances can be absorbed into and distributed within the human body, and how they are absorbed and distributed depends on the nature of their physical and chemical properties. The primary routes of absorption into the body are via the respiratory system, the skin, or oral ingestion into the digestive tract. Absorbed chemical substances are then distributed to several tissues and organs in the body.

Gene mutations in DNA and Onset of cancer cell

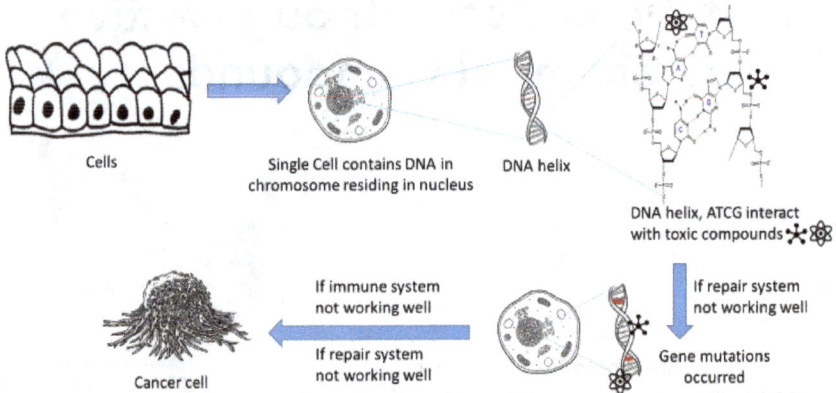

Cells

Single Cell contains DNA in chromosome residing in nucleus

DNA helix

DNA helix, ATCG interact with toxic compounds

If immune system not working well

If repair system not working well

Cancer cell

If repair system not working well

Gene mutations occurred

The absorbed chemical substances are metabolized within organs and tissues via biochemical reactions in the body, forming their metabolites. Some activated toxic metabolites formed will continuously interact with micro-molecules in the cells, causing irritation, inflammation, or even binding to cellular proteins or DNA molecules. In the worst-case scenario, gene mutations would occur in the DNA molecules, leading to the onset of cancer cells when the repairing system or defense mechanism is not working properly in the body.

A tumor consists of a heterogeneous mixture of millions of cells. A fraction of the mixture is equipped to leave the primary tumor. Cancer cells from a tumor can disseminate via blood vessels, invade the surrounding organs or distant organs, and begin to sprout and flourish there.

Proliferation of cancer cells and metastasis

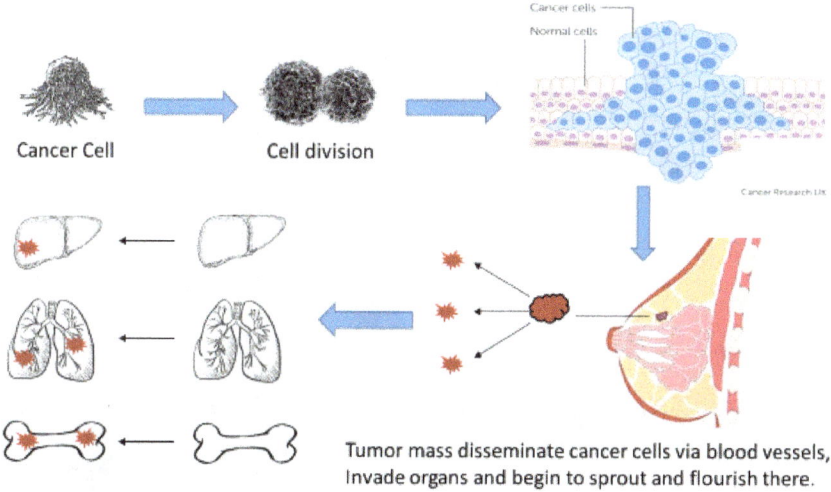

Cancer Cell   Cell division

Tumor mass disseminate cancer cells via blood vessels,
Invade organs and begin to sprout and flourish there.

Metastasis is the result of a pathological relationship between a cancer cell and its environment. Favored sites for cancer metastasis include the liver, the bones, the lungs, and the brain.

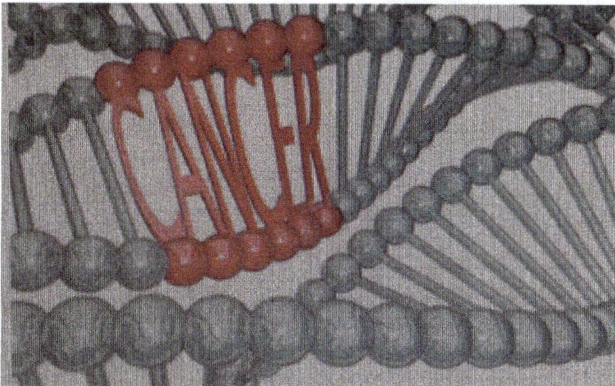

Introduction

The Average Longevity of Mankind

In 1914, the average life expectancy in the US was about 47 years. Before World War II, the average lifespan in most underdeveloped countries was below 40 years.

Studies show that the short lifespans of the past can be primarily attributed to bacteria, either via direct infection of the pathogen from unsanitary living or from infections spread by sickened patients. The absence of scientific, medical, or public knowledge of the bacteria and its corresponding infectious diseases allowed for many deaths.

In 1928, the first antibiotic, penicillin, was discovered in the United Kingdom, and it effectively fought against some bacterial infections. From 1940 onwards, several more effective antibiotics such as sulfonamide, tetracycline, and streptomycin were developed. Through the last several decades, many kinds of antibiotics and vaccines have been developed to fight against a wide range of infectious diseases. With these advances in science and medical technology, as well as better sanitation and hygiene care in daily life, the life expectancy of humans has risen sharply.

Despite these wonderful scientific and technological advances that were made in the last several decades, cancer still asserts itself as a formidable challenge to human life today.

Cancer Research and Development

Studies on cancer and cancer treatment began in the early 1900s. As the level of scientific knowledge and medical technology available to treat cancer at that time was very primitive, the diagnosis of cancer was equivalent to a death penalty.

In early 1900s, X-ray technology was introduced and became the core medical technology for dealing with cancer. At that time, when a cancer lump was found through an X-ray scan, there were only two treatment options available — either removing the cancer lump by surgery or burning the cancer lump with X-ray beams.

At the turn of the 21st century, technologies for cancer treatment evolved rapidly as experience with cancer treatment and scientific knowledge accumulated. The principal strategy for cancer treatment was, and still is today, to utilize drugs that are cytotoxic enough to kill growing cancer cells, also known as chemotherapy.

Chemotherapy drugs are effective in destroying bulks of cancer cells at a time. However, rapidly dividing non-cancer cells can be also damaged by chemotherapy as chemotherapy drugs are designed to target any cells that are in the process of dividing into new cells.

Today, cancer patients have alternative options to chemotherapy. Rather than relying on chemotherapy drugs that massively target all dividing cells including normal cells, patients can now opt for new anti-cancer drugs that are designed to eradicate only cancer cells by targeting specific molecules existing in cancer cells. In addition to these anti-cancer-targeted drugs, there are innovative new anti-cancer drugs being developed such as CART-T Cells, programmed cell death protein 1 (PD-1)/programmed cell death ligand 1 (PD-L1) inhibitors, virus vaccines, and anti-body drug conjugate (ADC) drugs.

However, cancer cells still can escape from the attack of newly developed anti-cancer drugs by avoiding the sphere of toxicity of the drugs or finding new pathways to survive, eventually metastasizing to different organs and tissues.

Due to the complexity of cancer types and their pathways for survival and proliferation, cancer researchers still have a long way to go before a comprehensive understanding of the underlying mechanisms of cancer can be achieved. However, cancer should be able to be classified as a curable disease someday in the future, owing to tremendous efforts of scientists in developing a variety of new drugs and technologies.

Initial Reaction to Cancer Diagnosis

Given the fatal outcome of cancer, panic is the common initial reaction from a person diagnosed with cancer. With lack of knowledge about the nature of cancer and treatment options, most patients become overwhelmed with anxiety. Then, patients are trying to learn about the cancer and their future with the disease. However, it is not easy for cancer patients to gain a comprehensive understanding of cancer overnight. Information about the disease is scattered throughout many different resources, and the information is also complex and difficult for ordinary people to understand.

Common initial questions that patients have upon receiving a cancer diagnosis are as follows.

1. What kinds of cancer drugs or treatments are available to cure my cancer?
2. How effective are current medical care and technology options for curing my cancer?

3. How long do I need to undergo chemotherapy?
4. When can I stop the cancer treatment?
5. How much is the cost of treatment?
6. Do I have a chance of winning the fight against cancer?
7. How long will I be able to live?

Road Map for Cancer Patients

There is something very important that cancer patients should know about and doctors should educate cancer patients before starting cancer treatments.

Of importance is a road map for cancer patients to go through such as tests and treatment needed like biopsies, manipulation of bone marrow tissues, radiotherapy and chemotherapy. And the road map should include explanation about following work after medical treatments have been completed, and how to manage the rest of life. Patients should be made aware of the physical stress and level of pain they may have to go through as part of their informed decision-making for treatment options. Patients should be mentally prepared with a realistic expectation of what the treatment outcome would be like. This means that doctors should provide patients with a road map of the processes involved and rationale for treatments. This information should be thoroughly reviewed with patients to ensure that they have a clear understanding of what lies ahead.

Providing information for patients to understand the how, what, and why of each step of the treatment plan, as well as a realistic range of possible outcomes, is important in preventing patients from feeling burdened with an incurable disease. Information can help patients reduce anxiety and give patients a greater sense of ownership in their treatment process. This sense of ownership is imperative to a positive attitude for patients fighting cancer.

In summary, upon diagnosis of cancer, doctors should provide patients with a detailed explanation of the stage and condition of the cancer and the treatment options available. Conversely, cancer patients should try to learn about anti-cancer treatment options, the entirety of the respective treatment processes, expected outcomes of the treatments, and expected post-treatment lifestyle before going through cancer treatments.

Guiding Questions to Better Understand the Cancer

The following questions serve to guide readers in gaining a better understanding of cancer and the tools available for cancer treatments.

Why and how do people get cancer? Can it be prevented? What is the difference between cancer and other diseases? What should we do if cancer is diagnosed or has progressed? How can we treat it? At which point does the cancer treatment end?

Through several chapters, this book explains some important concepts about cancer such as the onset of cancer, surgery, radiotherapy, chemotherapy, recovering from cancer, the recurrence of cancer, rehabilitation programs, and pathways to the end of life. This book will also provide a short introduction to toxicology so that readers can be aware of the potential risks of exposure to chemical substances as well as ways to prevent cancer in our day-to-day life.

The following are key topics to be explained in the chapters of this book:

1. Toxicology and risk of cancer
2. Types of cancer and their classification
3. Understanding anti-cancer treatments
4. Understanding tumor surgery and chemotherapy
5. Post-chemotherapy management
6. Clinical trials for cancer patients
7. Should I participate in a clinical trial? Pros and cons of clinical trials
8. Excessive medical treatment
9. Risk/benefit/cost assessment
10. Cancer risk, sign or symptom, and detection
11. Quality of life
12. Hospice care
13. Contemplation of death

Learning about Cancer and Treatments

Armed with a Ph.D. in Toxicology and substantial experience in the clinical development of oncology drugs, the author would like to share some useful information and scientific knowledge with readers, especially cancer patients. Most of the information in this book is supported by the findings of published scientific studies. The book is aimed at arming readers with knowledge about various aspects of cancer and guiding cancer patients through the treatment and recovery process. As cancers are very much diverse and complex, it is hoped that this book presents the information surrounding various types of cancers clearly and simply, so that ordinary people can understand cancers easily and manage their life with cancer effectively.

Cancer should be treated with cancer specialists who are experienced with the specific type of cancer. Furthermore, to obtain better results from cancer treatment, cancer patients should also acquire some basic knowledge about cancer and treatments.

The method and process involved in treating a cancer patient will vary, depending upon the cancer's type, stage, and location when it is diagnosed. Early stage cancer is relatively easy to treat with simple surgery and, if needed, followed by some anti-cancer drug therapy. However, medium-stage, late-stage, or fast-growing cancers are more difficult to deal with.

Doctors working in public hospitals in many countries are often constrained by the hospital system, policies, and limited resources while trying to take care of many patients. Physicians in a large hospital may be allocated only about 5 minutes for each patient per visit. Under such working conditions and resource constraints, it will be difficult for cancer patients to expect good quality medical services from doctors.

After being discharged from the hospital, the situation can become worse for cancer patients as they would be left alone to fight the cancer by themselves. And there seems to be no appropriate guidance available for patients who have been discharged. Cancer patients discharged from the hospital may try doing anything to improve their health such as searching for newly developed drugs, alternative therapies, natural remedies, functional foods, and supplementary care.

So, how should patients fight cancer on his or her own? There is no easy or right answer to this question. To cope with cancer more effectively, we should learn about cancer, cancer treatments, types of anti-cancer drugs, and how to manage the life with cancer. The book also discusses about the excessive medical treatment versus the quality of life in terminal stage cancer patients, and their passage to the final exit.

All Human Beings will Eventually become Patients Suffering Disease

Life is a journey of birth, growing, aging, illness, and death. All human beings experience certain kinds of disease before death, but each individual's way of living and dying is very much different. Accordingly, the onset and progress of cancer are very complex and difficult to deal with, due to the complexity of cancer disease combined with the biological diversity of each individual.

Until perfect medical technologies that cure cancer are available, all cancer patients will have to continue dealing with personal challenges to cope with the complex disease. It is important to make sure that cancer patients get the right support to cope with the long-term difficulties such as physical, emotional, financial, and other problems that cancer can inflict.

The author strives to use layman terms to explain the various scientific aspects of cancer from its onset, surgery, treatment, recurrence, and rehabilitation, and ultimately touching on death. The author goes beyond science to discuss the other aspects of cancer treatment — the quality of life and the farewell to life — that are also important realities that cancer patients should contemplate.

It is the author's wish that by reading and understanding the information in this book, cancer patients can be better equipped both mentally and emotionally so that they may undergo cancer treatments more smoothly and continue maintaining a decent quality of life.

Contents

1 Toxicology and Toxic Substances in Daily Life

What is Toxicology?

Toxicology is a branch of biology, chemistry, and medicine that is concerned with the study of the adverse effects of chemicals on living organisms. It also focuses on the harmful effects of chemical, biological, and physical agents in biological systems and strives to determine the extent of damage in living organisms.

Factors that influence toxicity include the dosage, route of exposure, species, age, sex, environment, and individual characteristics. The goal of toxicity assessment is to identify the adverse effects of a substance. The level of adverse effects mainly depends on the following three factors: (i) the routes of exposure (oral, inhalation, or dermal), (ii) the dosage of substances, and (iii) the duration of exposure — acute or chronic.

A toxicologist is a scientist or medical professional who specializes in the study of symptoms, mechanisms, treatments, and detection of toxins and venoms.

What is a Toxic Substance?

It would not be an exaggeration to say that all substances in our world are toxic. Any substance, even those regarded as pure and mild, can be toxic depending on the substance exposure conditions including how much or how long the exposure was, which routes or which sites the substance entered or passed through, and to whom the substance was exposed.

In our daily lives, we are exposed to various substances from the environment and the many household goods we use. Most of the time, we do not recognize or respond to the substances we are exposed to because the exposure duration is transient and the exposed dosage is very low. However, when exposure frequency is high and chronic, our body will react to the substance sometime later in the future. The level of response to certain toxic substances can vary depending on the exposure conditions and the individual traits of exposed persons.

The over-the-counter (OTC) or prescription drugs we consume always contain two different sides. One side produces the efficacy of the drug while the other side leads to side effects (toxicities). Efficacy and toxicity exist like two sides of a coin, and depending on the dose and frequency of the drug intake, the body will respond differently. Thus, the toxicity of any substance depends on how we are exposed to it.

Toxic Substances Hidden in Daily Life

The surrounding environment, including the ubiquitous household goods we use every day, regularly expose us to chemical substances. Usually, our bodies, when healthy, do not respond sensitively or quickly when exposed to these chemical substances as their concentration is not substantially high and the exposure time is transient.

However, when exposure to a certain chemical substance becomes chronic, even at low concentrations, the body may respond to the chemical substance adversely and manifest as irritations, inflammations, allergies, or even gene mutations of DNA.

When people are weakened by illness which results in poorer immunity, the reactions to external toxic substances will become more significant and can lead to more serious illnesses.

If someone gets exposed to an excessive amount of toxic chemical substance that is acutely absorbed into the body, this is almost certainly serious and will require urgent medical support.

People should be aware and cautious of the potential harms that arise from exposure to chemical substances in the environment, their household goods, and the things they may take for granted in everyday life.

Examples of Prolonged Exposure to Toxic Substances

The following are major substances that harbor toxicities to which people are exposed in daily life:

1. Tobacco cigarette smoking or indirect smoking (second-hand smoke);
2. Alcohol drinking;
3. Inhalation of polluted air (especially particulate matters smaller than 10 micrometers), which may be caused by factors ranging from plants to cars in metro cities;
4. Consumption of various food additives and preservatives in food products such as flavored drinks, barbecue-smoked red meat, and heavily salted fish; and

5. Sensitizing surfactants contained in detergents, anti-bacterial ingredients, anti-mold ingredients, environmental hormones released from various petrochemical products, insecticides, and pesticide residues.

Absorption, Distribution, Metabolism, and Excretion of Chemical Substances

The various chemical substances we are exposed to have their own unique characteristics with different patterns of absorption and distribution into the human body, depending on the nature of their physical and chemical properties.

The primary routes that chemical substances get absorbed into the body are via the respiratory system, the skin, and oral ingestion into the digestive tract. Absorbed chemical substances are then distributed to several organs and tissues within the body. Next, the chemical substances are metabolized within these organs and tissues via biochemical reactions in the body. Lastly, the resulting metabolites will be excreted from the body via several biological pathways.

Metabolism of Toxic Substances and Reactions from the Human Body

Most responses to toxic substances happen during the metabolic processes that occur within the body. The response can be fast (acutely) or slow (gradually) or may even appear only after many long years of dormancy, like cancer.

These metabolic processes encompass a range of biochemical reactions that occur with various enzymes, chemical substances, and co-factors in the body. When some activated toxic metabolites are initially formed in the body, the metabolic processes will try to neutralize or detoxify the activated metabolites with various internal molecules such as anti-oxidants and enzymes.

When a positive protective balance exists between the activation of toxic metabolites and the detoxification of toxic metabolites, the body will not experience any adverse symptoms of toxicity. However, when people's immune systems are weakened or compromised, their detoxification processes work less effectively and they are likely to get sick from the activated toxic metabolites. These activated toxic metabolites will continuously interact with micro-molecules in the cells, causing irritation or inflammation, or even binding to cellular proteins or DNA molecules. Among these reactions, one of the worst forms of toxic-metabolite interaction are genetic mutations caused by DNA molecules, giving rise to oncogenes and further transformations into cancer cells.

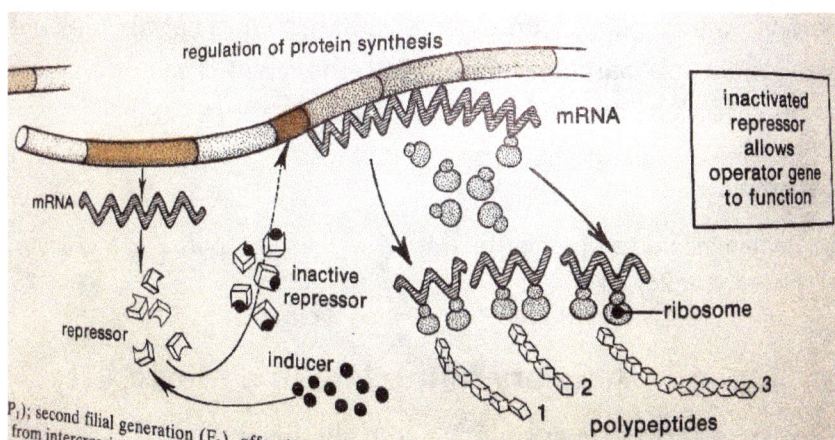

Picture of protein synthesis with DNA genes, mRNA, ribosomes, etc. from *Biochemistry, 3rd ed.* Lubert Stryer, W.H. Freeman and Company.

When the normal process of protein synthesis is interfered with by toxic metabolites, abnormal proteins get synthesized instead. These abnormally synthesized proteins can cause various types of diseases and trigger the transformation of normal cells into cancer cells.

Chapter 13 discusses how gene mutations are increasingly observed in people as they age. From DNA analyses, gene mutations were found in about 10% of people older than 65 and about 20% of people older than 90.[1]

This data indicates that the higher risk of cancer onset is related to aging and this is due to more pre-cancer cells with mutated genes silently harboring in old people. A large amount of pre-cancer cells with mutated genes in elderly people is the result of long-term exposure to various types of toxic substances throughout the lifetime.

People usually do not sense or recognize the constant stress on their body that arises from the interaction of activated chemical substances with cellular molecules. However, when their defense mechanisms (immunity) and/or repairing capabilities are weakened at a particular time point, the silent disaster waiting to burst forth at the molecular level will be cancer cells.

Reference

1.   Benjamin Ebert and Janis Abkowitz. *New England Journal of Medicine*, November 26, 2014.

Mr. Onco — A Salary Man's Life in a Metro City

Exposures to toxic substance in daily life

Mr. Onco is a salary man who lives in a metropolitan city. He commutes to a company that is located in the downtown area to work. Let's take look at his lifestyle and what kinds of toxic substances he might be exposed to while living and working in the city.

Mr. Onco wakes up in the morning with a headache due to alcohol drinking the night before. He drinks a glass of cold water before going to the bathroom for a shower. He uses a bar soap and shampoo to clean his body, after which he thoroughly rinses off with water. Next, he styles his hair with hair gel and spray, applies cream lotion on his face, and sprays deodorant onto his body. After having a quick breakfast, he brushes his teeth with a good amount of toothpaste. Lastly, he puts on his suit and sprays some cologne before leaving the house.

He walks along the street for 10 minutes to take the bus and arrives at the office in 40 minutes. During his walk, he frequently inhales exhaust gas or fumes emitted by nearby vehicles.

He works from 9.00 am to 6.00 pm. During work hours, he drinks a few cups of coffee using disposable paper cups. He eats lunch with colleagues at a restaurant near the office which offers a wide variety of high calorie foods with tasty seasonings. In the evening he joins a course a dinner with business partners or hangs out with his colleagues drinking beer, wine, and sometimes strong liquor and smoking cigarettes.

He heads home by walking and riding on a bus through the smog-filled city. At home, he uses anti-bacterial soap for his evening shower and brushes his teeth with toothpaste containing fancy ingredients. Sometimes, he does dishwashing and the laundry using detergents and fragrant fabric conditioners. Mr. Onco places mothballs and insect repellents in the closets and drawers as well as chemical deodorants in the room. The windows are tightly sealed to keep the room temperature at a comfortable level and to prevent polluted air from entering the room.

This is a typical pattern how a single salaryman, Mr. Onco, lives and works in a metro city. This lifestyle is also common for many ordinary people living in highly urbanized areas.

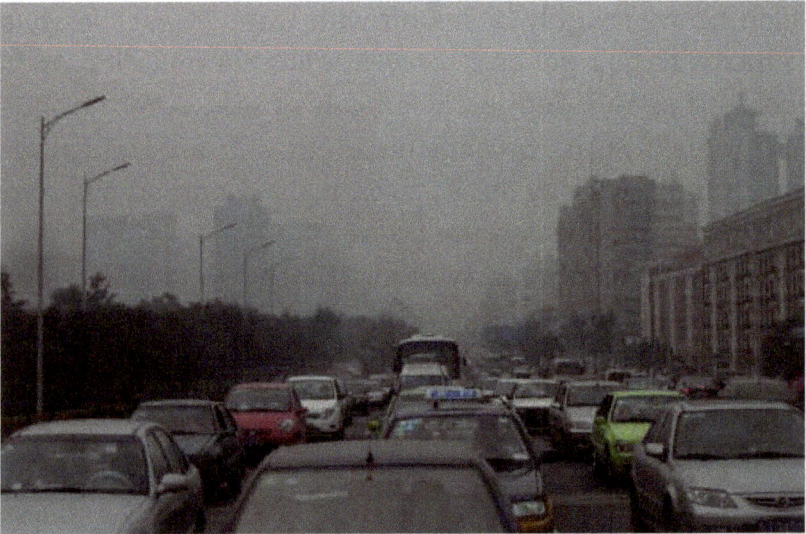

Air pollution and fumes in the city — picture from WHO (World Health Organization).

Let's find out in Chapter 2 what kinds of chemical substances Mr. Onco is exposed to in his daily life in the city.

Chapter 2

Toxic Substances and Biochemical Reactions in the Body

Toxic Chemical Substances that Mr. Onco is Exposed to, in his Daily Life

As seen in Chapter 1, there are numerous items containing chemical substances that Mr. Onco is exposed to every day. These include disposable paper cups, plastic cups, toilet paper, bar soap, shampoo, conditioner, shower gel, hair spray, perfume, deodorants, toothpaste, car exhaust fumes, smog, cigarette smoke, alcohol, high doses of caffeine, sugars in carbonated beverage, smoked or barbecued red meat, highly salted fish, various types of food additives, fine dust (particulate matters) from plants and construction, and possibly much more.

Regular exposure to the various types of chemical substances contained in these products can negatively impact our health.

Alcohol Consumption: The Body's Reaction to High Doses of Alcohol

People are exposed to alcohol (ethanol) when they drink alcoholic beverages such as liquor, beer, and wine. When swallowed, alcohol goes directly to the numerous cells and cell layers making up the stomach wall. When the mucosa of certain cell lines in the inner stomach wall are exposed to an intolerably high dosage of alcohol, the cells will get wounded and can die eventually.

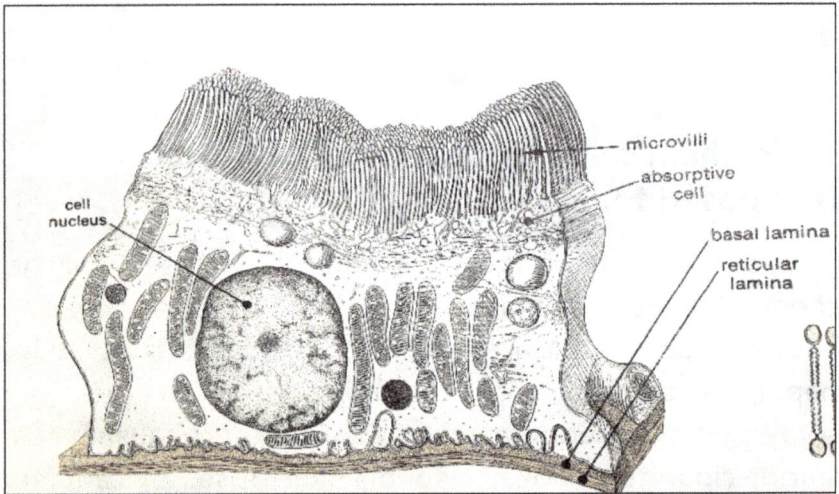

Picture of stomach wall with cells and layers. (From *Mellnoi's Illustrated Dictionary*. The Williams & Wilkins Company.)

When the cells are wounded, hormones and growth factors are released to treat the wounded cells. The released hormones and growth factors also flow into the pool of reserved cells to help restore parts of the stomach wall. The pool of reserved cells under or between the layer of the stomach wall responds to the signals from hormones and growth factors, producing new cells to replace the damaged or dead cells. Usually the stomach cells will quickly respond to the emergency and effectively recover and protect the stomach wall with new cells.

However, frequent consumption of high doses of alcohol would cause chronic damage to the stomach cells. This unhealthy and oftentimes painful situation will require new cells to heal the wounded areas. New cells are produced by a kind of cell manufacturing operation with numerous cell divisions requiring DNA/gene replications.

As more cell divisions occur, the chance of interactions between cellular molecules including DNA and external chemical substances increases. Frequent interactions of DNA/genes and cellular molecules with external active chemical substances may cause a higher probability of gene mutations, leading to the production of abnormal cells. The abnormal cells produced due to gene mutations may transform into cancer cells.

Intolerable doses of alcohol will cause initial damage to the stomach followed by secondary damage to the liver. Alcohol metabolites formed in the liver will cause stress to liver cells. When the stress from alcohol metabolites persists for a long period of time, it will lead to alcohol-related fatty liver, liver sclerosis, and finally liver cancer.

In addition, excessive alcohol drinking also causes damage to other organs in the body including the brain. The brain cells can also be destroyed by a large amount of alcohol ingestion.

The following is a summary of the links between alcohol drinking and cancer risk as documented by published studies.

Alcohol is causally associated with various types of cancers, and the greatest risks are observed with heavy, long-term ingestion of alcohol. Even a modest ingestion of alcohol may increase cancer risk. Cancer risk from alcohol consumption has been observed consistently regardless of the specific type of alcoholic beverage (e.g., beer, wine, or other liquors) consumed.[1]

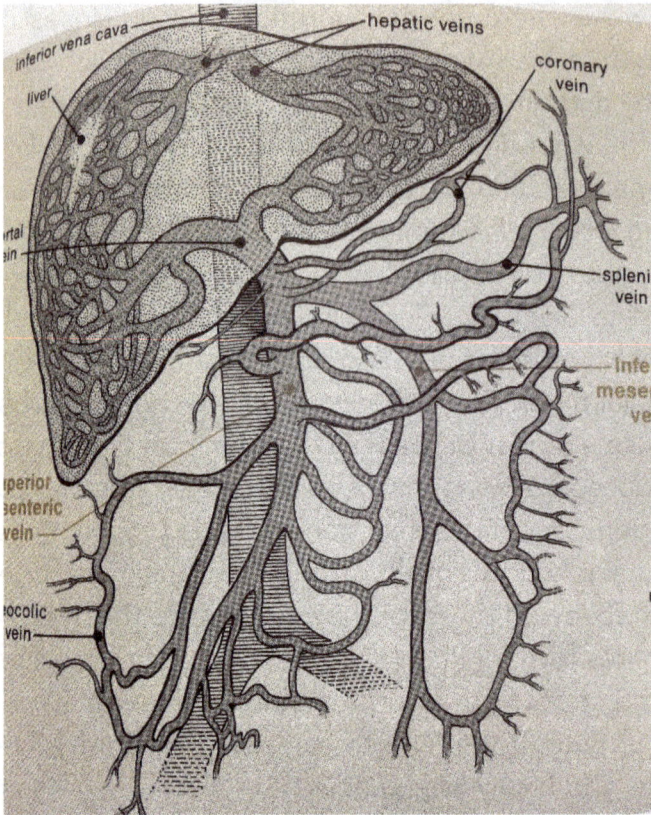

Picture of cross-flowing blood vessels inside and outside the liver.

Alcohol is metabolized and eliminated from the body by alcohol dehydrogenase. During the metabolic process, alcohol (ethanol) is oxidized first to acetaldehyde and then to acetate. Acetaldehyde is mutagenic by binding to DNA and proteins in the body.[2]

Prolonged alcohol-induced oxidative stress can result in chronic tissue inflammation via the CYP2E1 pathway.[3] Alcohol drinking affects circulating hormones in the body like androgens and estrogens, which can contribute to breast cancer.[3] Alcohol ingestion is also associated with lower folate concentrations in the body which is related to the etiology of colon cancer.[4]

When alcohol is absorbed into body cells, CYP2E1 enzymes are sharply induced. CYP2E1 enzymes metabolize various types of xenobiotics or carcinogenic compounds into more bioactive forms, causing toxic binding to DNA or proteins.

References

1. IARC Working Group on the Evaluation of Carcinogenic Risks to Humans. Personal habits and indoor combustions, in *A Review of Human Carcinogens*. Lyon, France, 2009.
2. Pöschl G, Seitz HK. Alcohol and cancer. *Alcohol Alcoholism* **39**:155–165, Crossref, Medline, 2004.
3. Van't Veer P, Kampman E. *Food, Nutrition, Physical Activity, and the Prevention of Cancer: A Global Perspective*. Washington, DC, World Cancer Research Fund/American Institute for Cancer Research, 2007.
4. World Cancer Research Fund/American Institute for Cancer Research: Food, Nutrition, Physical Activity, and the Prevention of Cancer: A Global Perspective. Washington, DC, American Institute for Cancer Research, 2007.

Statement from the American Society of Clinical Oncology (ASCO) on alcohol and cancer prevention

According to the statement from ASCO issued in 2017, alcohol consumption is a contributing factor to cancer and excessive alcohol consumption can negatively affect cancer treatment. ASCO cites between 5% and

6% of new cancer cases and deaths globally as being directly attributable to alcohol consumption.[1] However, most people do not recognize alcohol consumption as a risk factor for cancer.

Reference

1. LoConte NK, Brewster AM, Kaur JS, *et al*. Alcohol and cancer: A statement of the American Society of Clinical Oncology. *J Clin Oncol* [epub ahead of print], 2017.

Smoking

When smoking a cigarette, lots of carcinogenic chemicals are inhaled and absorbed into the lungs. The representative carcinogens include benzo-pyrene, PAH (poly-aromatic hydrocarbon), formaldehyde, dioxin, arsenic, nitrosamine, and nicotine.

Toxic chemicals that are absorbed into the lungs are circulated and distributed to other tissues and organs. These chemicals are then processed, metabolized, and eventually excreted from the body. An important point to understand is that secondary and tertiary toxic metabolites can be formed by biochemical reactions during the metabolic processes in the body. Toxic metabolites formed in the body can penetrate cells and bind to DNA or other cellular molecules, causing abnormalities in the cells.

Cigarette smoking can cause not only lung cancers but also various other types of cancers in other organs and tissues in the body, as the carcinogenic toxic compounds and their metabolites formed get circulated via blood vessels to all parts of the body.

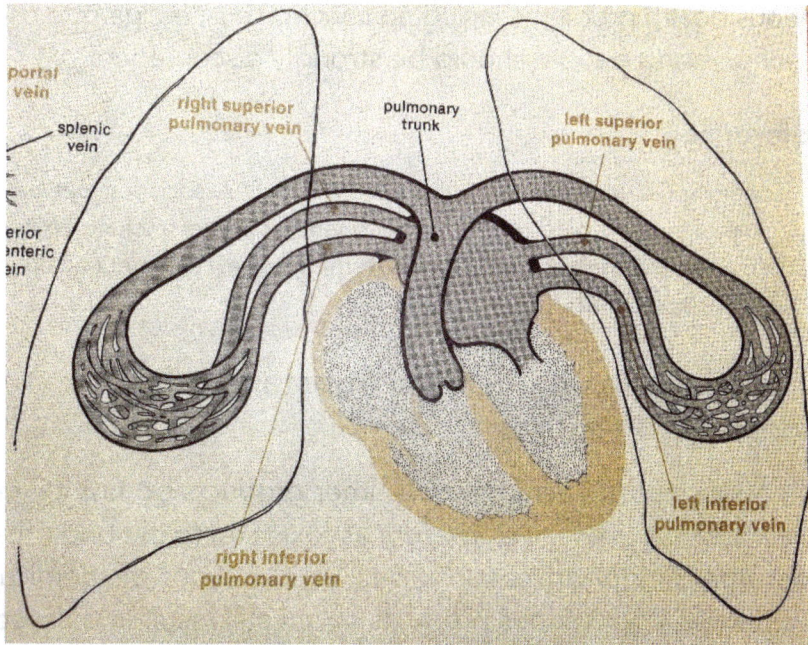

portal
vein

splenic
vein

right superior
pulmonary vein

pulmonary
trunk

left superior
pulmonary vein

erior
nteric
ein

left inferior
pulmonary vein

right inferior
pulmonary vein

Picture of Cross-flowing blood vessels through the lungs and heart. (From *Mellnoi's Ilustrated Medical Dictionary*. The Williams & Wilkins Company.)

E-Cigarettes versus Tobacco Smoking

A study[1] reported that e-cigarette use may lead to tobacco cigarette smoking in future. Young people aged 14 to 30 years who used e-cigarettes were 3.6 times more likely to smoke tobacco cigarettes later than those who never used e-cigarettes. This means that e-cigarettes are not merely a substitute for tobacco cigarettes but also present a strong risk factor for future smoking.

Like tobacco smoking, the evidence clearly shows that e-cigarettes, smokeless tobacco, and water pipes may also cause serious health problems including cancer. Thus, e-cigarette use among young people should be strongly discouraged.

Reference

1. Soneji S, Barrington-Trimis JL, Wills TA, *et al*. Association between initial use of e-cigarettes and subsequent cigarette smoking among adolescents and young adults: A systematic review and meta-analysis. *JAMA Pediatr* **171**:788–797, 2017.

Potentially Toxic Chemical Substances from Consumer Products

Although ingredients from consumer products do not cause quick adverse events (i.e., present as toxicities) to the body, the consumer's long-term exposure to various types of chemical substances from various products might still result in delayed health problems. Let's consider a few examples from the products we use every day.

- Tissue paper produced using unqualified recycled raw materials through poorly controlled manufacturing processes may induce irritation or cause infections to mucus membranes, as the paper may contain harmful germs and aggravating substances such as bleach. Inflammation can follow with mucosal infection from bacteria, further infecting the rest of the body.

- A shower space in a small apartment in a metro city is usually quite small and tightly sealed with a poor ventilation system. When people take a shower using, for instance, shower gels, hair shampoos, or conditioners containing various types of chemical ingredients, some of these ingredients are absorbed through the skin and scalp. Chemicals that are evaporated or aerosolized during the shower can be inhaled into the lungs. As discussed above, absorbed chemicals are distributed, metabolized, and later excreted from the body, but some metabolites formed in the body frequently interact with cellular molecules and can cause health-related problems.

- Synthetic laundry detergent, fabric softener, hair spray, hair gel, deodorant, and dishwashing detergent all contain various fragrance chemicals. Fragrances usually contain dozens of chemical ingredients in their formula. Although these fragrance chemical ingredients are often not acutely toxic, they can cause delayed adverse effects such as allergies. While some ingredients can be metabolized and easily excreted from the body, some other ingredients may bio-accumulate in the body for a long period of time. When non-biodegradable ingredients accumulate in the body for many years, biochemical reactions can occur later in the body, leading to delayed health problems.

The chemical ingredients used in consumer products are usually tested and assessed as safe-to-use with an exposure assessment tool before being released to the market. The typical toxicity tests conducted on consumer products include eye irritation, skin irritation, skin sensitization, inhalation safety, developmental toxicities, genotoxicity, and carcinogenicity. These tests are designed and conducted to ensure the safety of products, and the test methods used are typically in-vitro (laboratory tests), in-vivo (animal tests), and clinical tests mainly on human skin.

Global consumer product marketing companies rely on standard human safety programs to ensure the safety of products for consumer use. Safety data are generated with a certain safety margin versus a threshold value of toxicity. How-ever, concerns abound with these safety programs as current programs cannot possibly accommodate all conditions or situ-ations that may arise from consumer use and their exposure to various types of products. Furthermore, certain ingredients in consumer products may negatively impact consumers' health only after repeated use over the lifetime.

Many companies develop safe products based on sound science and stringent toxicological assessments on product formula. However, it is still difficult to eliminate health-related risks completely for consumers using these products. These difficulties arise from the different conditions under which con-sumers get exposed to the wide range of chemicals contained in various types of products, including each consumer's habits and practices.

Consumers may also face delayed health problems which occur only after many years of using multiple products. Hence, consumers should be vigilant about the safe use of a product by understanding its properties before use. Consumers should use products as guided, but also try to minimize exposure to the products' chemical ingredients as much as possible. Minimizing the exposure to chemical substances as much as possible should help to reduce the risk of delayed toxicity in a later part of life, since the risk of delayed toxicity can be proportional to the total amount of chemical substances that people have been exposed to, through the lifetime.

Environmental Hormones (Endocrine Disruptors)

The endocrine system is like a communication network in our body, coordinating and balancing a variety of body functions. There are several endocrine tissues in the body, such as the ovaries, testes, adrenal gland, pituitary gland, thyroid gland, and pancreas. They produce hormones and secrete them into the blood system, organs, and tissues throughout the body.

Hormones work with tissues, organs, and the nervous system to control many crucial functions in the body, such as body energy levels, reproduction, growth and development, internal balance, and response to external stress.

There are many endocrine-disrupting chemicals that people are exposed to in day-to-day living. The chemical structures and activities of endocrine-disrupting chemicals interfere with hormonal signals in the body, thereby causing health problems.

Endocrine disruptors, having similar structures to hormones in the body, can bind to receptors on cells and interfere with the usual binding activities of endogenous hormones. The normal signals from hormones will be disrupted and the body will not be able respond properly.[1]

Endocrine disruptors can be found in food and beverages, medicines, cosmetics, pesticides, plastic items, and many other common products. Examples of endocrine disruptors include diethylstilbestrol (DES — the synthetic estrogen), dioxin and dioxin-like compounds, polychlorinated biphenyls (PCBs), dichlorodiphenyltrichloroethane (DDT), bisphenol A (BPA), di(2-ethylhexyl) phthalate (DEHP), and perfluorinated compounds (PFC).[1]

Bisphenol A (BPA) is used in the production of polycarbonate plastics and epoxy resins. Di(2-ethylhexyl) phthalate (DEHP) is used in the manufacturing of food packaging, some children's products, and polyvinyl chloride (PVC) medical devices. Perfluorinated compounds (PFC), such as perfluorooc-tanic acid (PFOA) and perfluorooctanesulfonic acid (PFOS), can be released from disposable paper cups.[1]

Phytoestrogens are naturally found in plants and exhibit hormone-like activities. Examples of phytoestrogens are genistein and daidzein, which can be found in soy-derived products.

Various kinds of health problems can occur due to the absorption of endocrine disrupters into the body. In severe cases, endocrine disruptors can reduce the number of sperm in men and cause endometriosis or vaginal cancer in women.

Reference

1. National Toxicology Program's Report of the Endocrine Disruptors Low-Dose Peer Review 2001.

Food and Beverage

Coffee: Excessive drinking of coffee may result in insufficient sleep. Caffeine, especially at high doses, can cause arrhythmia in the hearts of some people.

Sugar: People often ingest food and beverages containing high amounts of sugar. In addition to such direct sugar intake, carbohydrate-based food also contributes to more sugar ingestion to the body. High amounts of sugar ingestion will lead to excessive body weight and obesity, resulting in various health risks.

Food additives: Food additives are chemical ingredients added to food for different purposes, such as coloring of food, shaping of food, supplementing nutrients, or prevention of food decay. Most processed food contains a lot of artificial additives. There are hundreds of food additives being used and they are classified as follows.

- Natural food additives or artificial synthetic chemical additives.
- Functional classifications: conservatives, disinfectants, anti-oxidants, colorants, bleach, seasoning, sweeteners, spices, enhancers, emulsifiers, skim, gum base, foam inhibitors, solvent, improvers, etc.

Every company that makes food products must comply with laws and regulations. Though there are certain guidelines and standard operating procedures to evaluate the safety of ingredients and product formulas, health-related issues can still occur due to poor quality food ingredients, contamination with impurities, or improper manufacturing processes for artificial food additives.

Cooked Food: People are exposed to various carcinogenic compounds from some types of cooked food such as barbecued red meat or salted fish. Carcinogenic compounds like benzopyrene, heterocyclic amines (HCA), polycyclic aromatic hydrocarbons (PAH), and nitrosamines are generated due to the incomplete combustion of meat protein and fat during charcoal burning. When salt (sodium nitrate) interacts with dimethylamine in the fish, carcinogenic N-nitrosoamine compounds are generated.

Smog in the City and Fine Dust

Long-term exposure to fine dust (particulate matter) from smog can lead to serious diseases in people. The diseases caused by particulate matter include stroke, ischemic heart disease, chronic obstructive pulmonary disease (COPD), and lung cancer. Fine dust is a pollutant that is mainly produced from power plants, cars, and manufacturing plants when fossil fuels are burned. These various types of pollutants circulating as chemical substances and ionic compounds can be inhaled into the lungs and distributed all over the body.

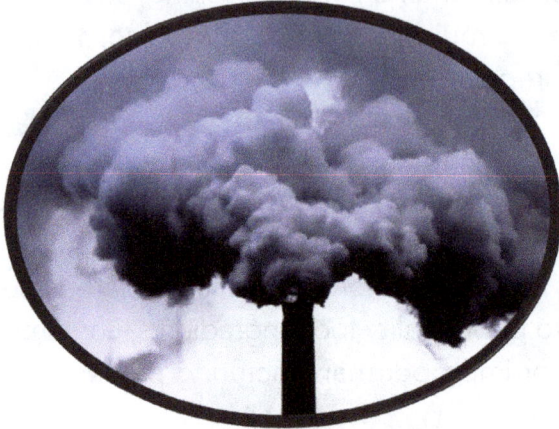

Classification of Fine Dust (Particulate Matter)

- PM-10 (Particulate Matter < 10 μm): particle size less than 10 microns
- PM-2.5 (Particulate Matter < 2.5 μm): particle size less than 2.5 microns

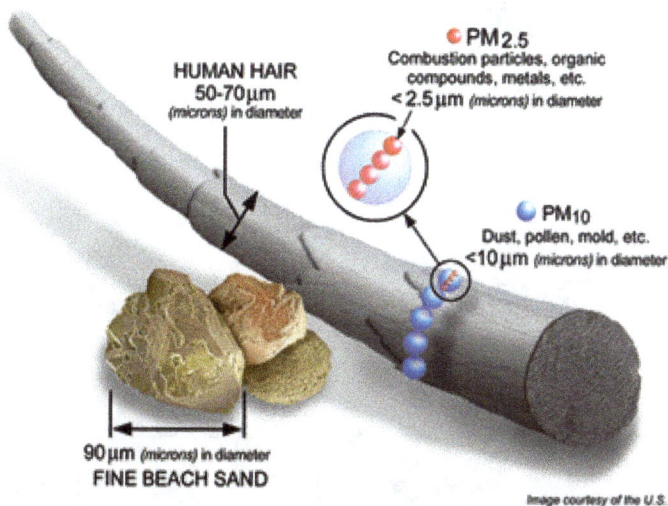

Picture showing the size of PM 2.5 and PM 10 versus the size of sand and hair.

Large dust particles can be filtered out when they pass through the branches of lung tubes before reaching the alveolar cells where a network of blood capillaries surrounds the alveoli sac. However, miniscule fine dust (e.g., PM-10), which are not easily agglomerated in nature, can directly infiltrate into the alveolar cells.

In other words, the smaller the size of fine dust particles, the harder it is to prevent their direct penetration into alveolar cells, leading to respiratory diseases or other impairments of the body's immune function.

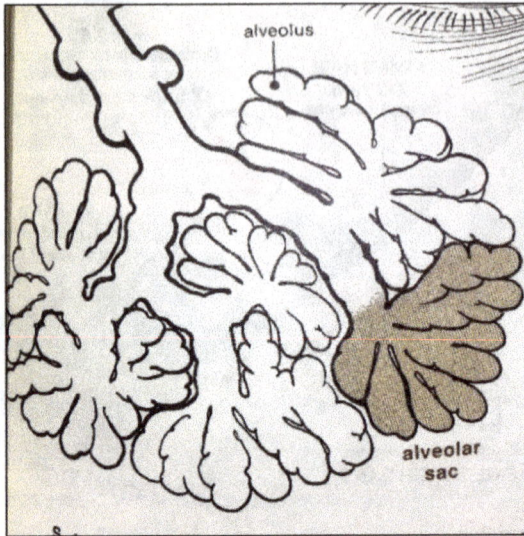

Picture of Alveolus — a basic unit of the lungs which is present in the alveola sac. From *Mellnoi's Illustrated Medical Dictionary*. The Williams & Wilkins Company.)

Fine dust bound with nitric ions or sulfuric ions can oxidize to form nitric oxides or sulfuric oxides, which can then infiltrate into the alveola cells. These compounds cause inflammation in the cells and tissues, resulting in health conditions such as bronchitis, asthma, COPD, and heart arrhythmia. In addition, they can stimulate white blood cells to inflame the walls of blood vessels, resulting in serious diseases such as arteriosclerosis, myocardial infarction, and stroke.

A study investigated the relationship between air pollution and mortality rates in adults living in six cities in the United States from 1974 to 2009. The study found that reduction of PM-2.5 at the rate of 2.5 μg/m^3 annually was correlated with 3.5% reduction in the mortality rate. In addition, longevity increased by 2.7 years from the 1980s to the 1990s. It was estimated that an increase of PM-2.5 by 10 μg/m^3 is associated with an increase in the mortality rate by 1.1%. Taken together, these indicate that air that is heavily polluted with fine dust is significantly related to the outbreak of disease and increased mortality rates in humans.

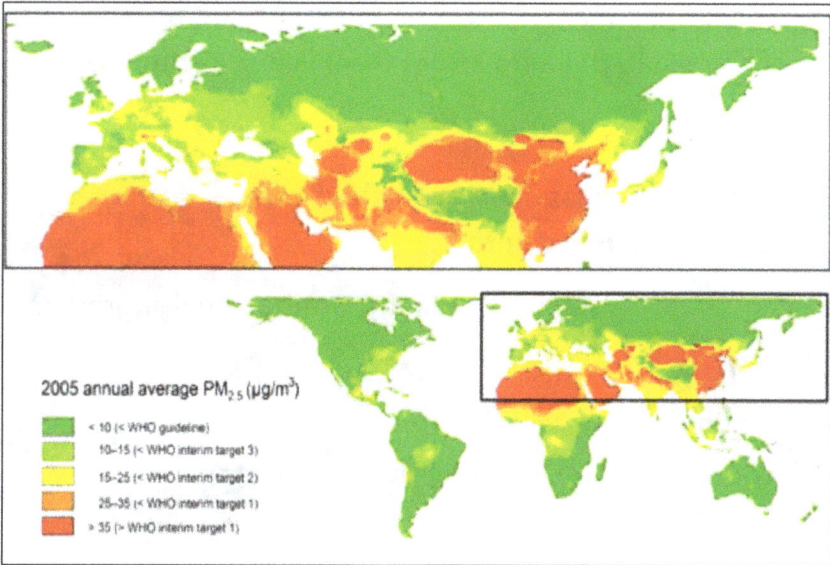

2005 annual average PM$_{2.5}$ (µg/m^3)

< 10 (< WHO guideline)
10–15 (< WHO interim target 3)
15–25 (< WHO interim target 2)
25–35 (< WHO interim target 1)
> 35 (> WHO interim target 1)

World map showing the areas of pollution with fine dust. Red colored areas indicate the heaviest levels of fine dust pollution. (Reference: World Health Organization.)

Asbestos

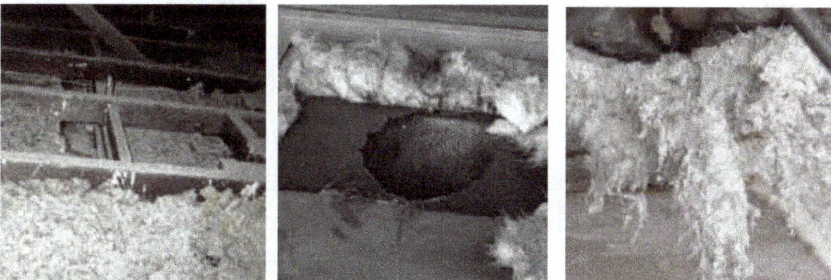

Many years ago, asbestos was widely used as insulation material in house or building construction. Some asbestos could still be left inside some old houses or buildings today. The particle size of asbestos is 1/5,000th of a hair's thickness and can directly infiltrate into lung cells and tissues. Lung cancer and pulmonary disease can occur from the infiltration of asbestos into the lung after 20–40 years. It is truly a silent killer.

Toxicity of Antibacterial Ingredients in Consumer Products

Examples of products containing antibacterial ingredients include:

- Kitchen detergents
- Deodorants or textile deodorant products
- Soap
- Shower gel
- Toothpaste products containing anti-microbial ingredients

Consumers use a variety of antibacterial products in daily life. On the surface, anti-microbial products seem to benefit the health of consumers by killing harmful germs. But products containing antibacterial ingredients may not be truly helpful in the prevention of diseases compared to the ordinary products in the same category.

Consumers can be misled by attractive commercial advertisements that take advantage of consumers' fear of the threat of bacterial infection. Consumer product marketing companies are competitively developing and marketing various types of antibacterial products with a bigger spectrum of antibacterial activities, which may be beneficial in killing bacteria but can also be harmful to health.

Some antibacterial ingredients from products can be absorbed into the body via the skin, mouth, or respiratory tract. For example, the ingredients of certain toothpaste products can be ingested or absorbed while we are brushing our teeth. There are several types of products containing antibacterial chemicals sold in the market, such as antibacterial soap, shower gel, detergents, fabric deodorants, dust mite repellents, anti-mold sprays, and insect repellents.

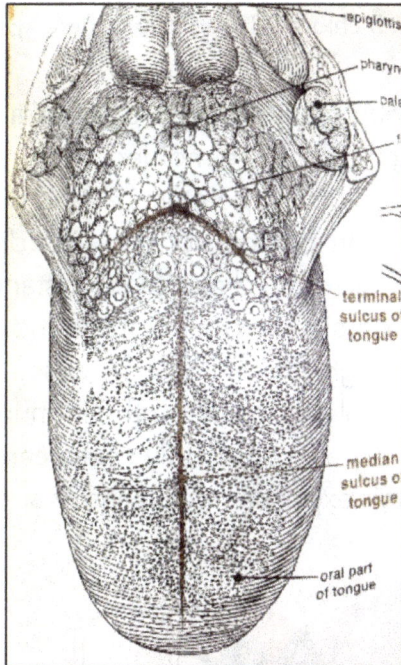

Picture of the tongue and throat. From *Mellnoi's Illustrated Medical Dictionary*. The Williams & Wilkins Company.)

Antibacterial Ingredients Used in Soap and their Toxicities

Triclosan is an antibacterial ingredient which has been widely used in the making of antibacterial soap. Triclosan is used alone or mixed together with trichlorocarbanilide in the soap formula to produce a synergy that kills bacteria more effectively.

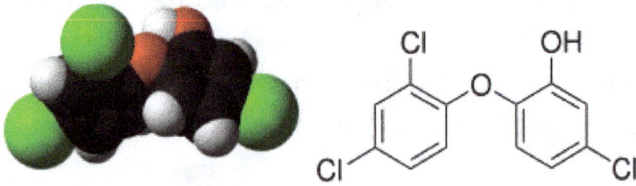

Triclosan: 5-chloro-2-(2,4-dichlorophenoxy)phenol.

During the soap manufacturing process, antibacterial soap scraps containing triclosan are molded into the shape of soap. When subjected to high temperatures during the manufacturing process, triclosan can be transformed into different types of chemicals such as dioxin or dioxin-like substances.

Dioxins are persistent pollutants found in the environment. Dioxins are highly toxic and can cause reproductive and developmental problems, damage the immune system, interfere with hormones, and ultimately cause cancer. Consumers should reduce their exposure to dioxins or similar substances.

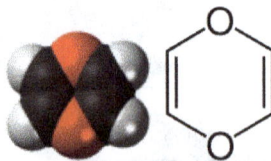

1,4-Dioxin.

What is the Difference between Antibacterial Soap and Regular Soap?

What kind of benefits can antibacterial soap give us compared to regular soap? Do antibacterial soaps really have superior germ-killing efficacy in comparison to regular soaps?

A laboratory test that was performed to compare the difference in antibacterial efficacy between antibacterial soap and regular soap when washing hands, and no difference was found. Another test was conducted to compare the antibacterial efficacy between washing hands with antibacterial soap and washing hands with just water. As expected, washing hands with antibacterial soap showed superior antibacterial efficacy compared to washing hands with water. Likewise, regular soap showed superior antibacterial efficacy compared to washing hands only with water.

There are commercial advertisements promoting the use of antibacterial products with the tagline "99.9% removal of bacteria." Such advertisements try to take advantage of consumers' emotional concerns about bacteria-transmitted disease. However, it is not certain if such commercial messages are really based on valid scientific data. Washing our hands with regular bar soaps should be good enough for the removal of dirt, fatty materials, and germs and bacteria. The sanitization efficacy of regular soap does not appear to be different from antibacterial soap.

Antibacterial Ingredient Triclosan and Liver Cancer

In November 2014, Dr. Robert H. Tukey (University of California, San Diego School of Medicine) published a study in the

Proceedings of the National Academy of Sciences on triclosan, which is used in many household goods including toothpaste and detergent products.

Dr. Tukey's research team conducted a toxicity test on triclosan with a group of mice and found that the mice developed liver tissue fibrosis and liver cancer after being exposed to triclosan for 6 months, which is equivalent to 18 years in humans. In addition, some of the mice also developed kidney tissue fibrosis.[1]

Triclosan is easily detected in the environment as it is widely used in many consumer products. Triclosan has been found in 75% of consumers' bodies and in the breast milk of 95% of breastfeeding mothers. Previous studies on products containing triclosan have warned pregnant women about the problems that triclosan can cause to fetal development. The study report also issued a warning that long-term exposure to triclosan may cause liver cancer in humans.[1]

Like triclosan, many other chemical ingredients from consumer products can be absorbed into the body. Some chemical ingredients can be detected in the blood after certain household products are used, such as toothpaste, shower gel, shampoo, conditioner, and spray-type products.

Certain chemical substances that are absorbed will be metabolized in the body. The chemicals and metabolites formed in the body can induce toxicities, starting from irritation, allergic reactions, or chronic health problem if they persistently remain within the body.

Reference

1. Robert H. Tukey, UC San Diego, School of Medicine. The proceedings of National Academy of Sciences, November 17, 2014.

A Simple Life to Avoid Exposure to Potential Toxic Substances

There are many regulatory guidelines in place to control the use of certain chemicals and ingredients in consumer products. Companies selling household products are responsible for the safety of their products by complying with the laws and regulatory guidelines of each country. In addition to legal and regulatory compliance, major global companies also operate their own safety assessment programs based on sound science and technology. Each product from these companies should be marketed only after safety assessments have been done to ensure that they can be safely used by consumers.

However, it is important for consumers to know that people are exposed to chemical substances everywhere from the surrounding environment, in addition to chemical substances from household products. This means that a safety program for each single product is not sufficient to help us avoid the risk of exposure to various chemicals from various types of products and other toxic substances in the environment. Since people are exposed to numerous chemical substances every day, it would be difficult to complete an accurate safety assessment of all the multi-chemical substances we are exposed to in daily life, many of which are unknown to us.

If we were able to accurately conduct a safety assessment of all the toxic chemical substances we are exposed to every day, the result of this safety assessment would be quite different from the risk assessment done by a company on a single chemical ingredient or a product formula.

The probability of getting an illness is proportionate to the frequency and duration of exposure to toxic chemical substances. One study on elderly people showed a close relationship between exposure to toxic substances and the quantity of pre-cancer cells existing in the blood. It was found that DNA gene mutations in blood cells increased with age, with about 10% of people older than 65 and about 20% of people older than 90 having gene mutations.

Hence, to maintain a healthy life style is to try and minimize exposure to potential toxic chemical substances in daily life by (i) avoiding the use of unnecessary products containing fancy ingredients such as antibacterial agents, fragrances, and artificial additives, and (ii) staying away from areas with heavily polluted air or water.

Risks Associated with Regular Health Examinations

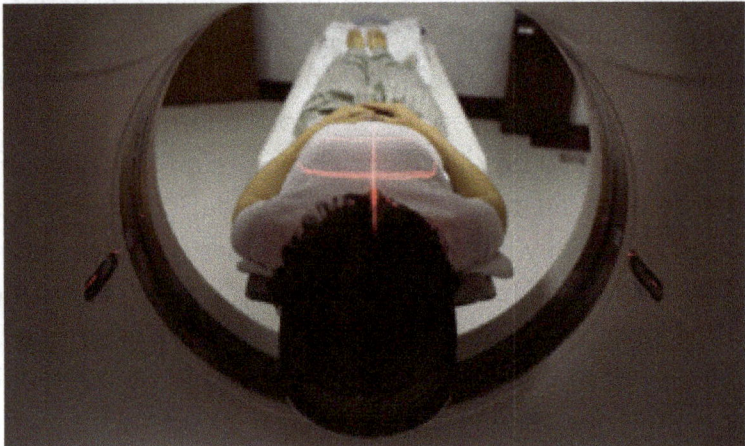

Picture of a computed tomography scan.

X-rays with strong energy beams can penetrate the body and produce pictures of internal body structures, which can then be viewed on photographic film or computer monitors. X-ray examinations are used to make accurate diagnoses of disease.

The scientific unit of measurement of a radiation dose is the millisievert (mSv). Other radiation dose measurement units include rad, rem, roentgen, sievert, and gray.

Different tissues and organs of the body have varying sensitivities to radiation. Thus, the risks associated with an X-ray scan and radiation will differ depending on the parts of the body that are exposed. Many people today are exposed to radiation via computed tomography (CT) scans and chest X-rays for health checks or disease treatment. Extended exposure to X-ray radiation will lead to greater health risks.

An article issued in August 2012 reported that exposure to radiation from CT scans in childhood is associated with higher risk of subsequent leukemia and brain tumors.[1] The data showed that the use of CT scans to deliver cumulative doses of about 50 mGy in children might triple the risk of leukemia, while doses of about 60 mGy might triple the risk of brain cancer.[1]

People should be aware of the risks of excessive health examinations using CT scans or X-rays.

Reference

1. The LANCET Volume 380, Issue 9840, 4–10 August 2012.

Cancer-related Bacteria and Viruses

In addition to minimizing exposure to toxic chemical substances in the environment, food, and consumer products, we also need to pay attention to cancer-causing bacteria and viruses. For example, the Helicobacter pylori bacteria can cause gastric cancer and Human Papilloma Virus (HPV) can cause cervical cancer and several other types of cancer.

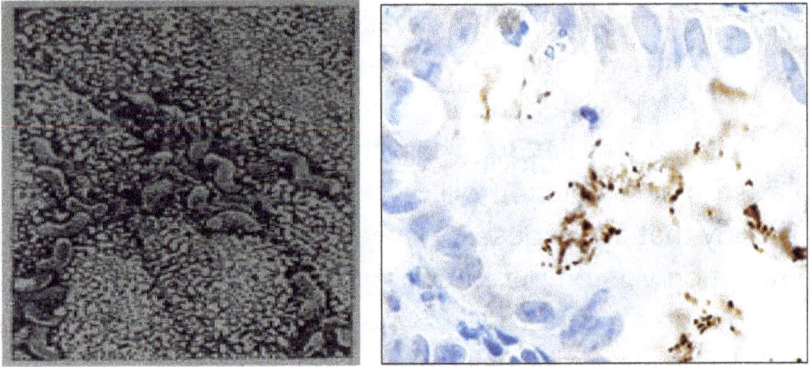

Picture of Helicobacter pylori bacteria (from Wikipedia).

Helicobacter pylori (*H. pylori*) bacteria was discovered in 1983. The bacteria live in the gastric mucous membrane of an infected person, secreting a variety of enzymes and toxins in the stomach. The body's immune system reacts against the toxins, thereby causing inflammation in the stomach which leads to gastritis, gastric ulcer, and duodenal ulcer. The risk of stomach cancer is doubled or tripled with the presence of *H. pylori* bacteria.

Infection is caused by the ingestion of food or water contaminated by feces containing *H. pylori* bacteria. It can also be transmitted from mouth to mouth. *H. pylori* bacteria infection was especially high among Asians in the past, but the current infection rate is significantly lowered due to improved sanitation and standards of living. *H. pylori* infection can be treated with a combination of antibiotics and anti-acids.

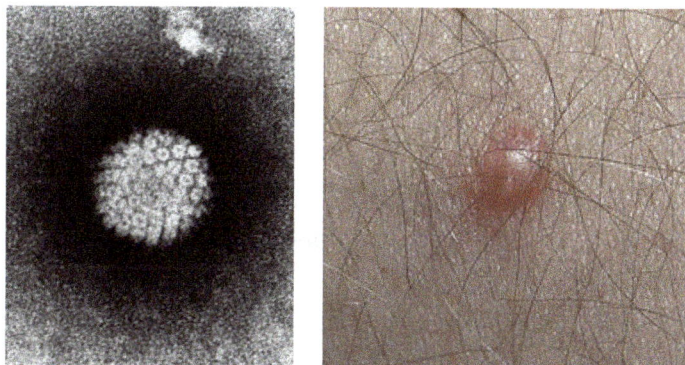

Human Papilloma Virus and Papilloma (pictures from Wikipedia).

According to the Center for Disease Control and Prevention (CDC), approximately 20 million people in the United States are infected with HPV, with 6.2 million new cases each year. There are more than 40 different types of HPV which infect organs, tissues, and the skin. HPV is transmitted through sexual contact with infected people, and HPV infection is not noticeable before the onset of clinical symptoms. Infected areas include the vulva, vagina, penis, and anus.

HPV is the major cause of cervical cancer and a large proportion of vaginal, vulvar, anal, penile, and head and neck (oral cavity and oropharynx) cancers. It was reported that 90% of papilloma infections were caused by HPV 6 and HPV 11 viruses, and about 70% of cervical cancers were caused by HPV 16 and HPV 18 viruses.

According to the CDC, American College of Obstetricians and Gynecologists, and the American Academy of Pediatrics, it is strongly recommended for both boys and girls to go for routine HPV vaccinations as they are at risk of developing HPV-related cancers. However, according to a study in 2014, vaccination rates remain low with only 40% of girls and 22%

of boys aged 13 to 17 completing the HPV vaccination series. Nonetheless, the Department of Health and Human Services has set a goal of reaching 80% vaccinations by 2020.

Some states in the US are trying to pass laws mandating that children must receive HPV vaccinations as part of school admissions, or that 11 and 12 year-old students must get HPV vaccinations before they can start 6th grade.

The HPV vaccine is the first vaccine that is successfully targeted against cancer. The HPV vaccine was approved in 2006 and is now available to children and adults, starting at the age of 9 up to age 26. There are two commercial HPV vaccines available in the market, namely Gardasil (Merck) and Cervarix (GSK).

Chapter 3

Factors Causing Disease and Factors Affecting Curing of Disease

In Chapter 2, we reviewed several examples of potential toxic substances in daily life that can cause adverse effects on health. Now, we will review some other key factors that affect health by categorizing them into three different groups: (1) internal factors, (2) intermediate factors, and (3) external factors.

Internal Factors

1. Genetics (e.g., genetic disease, sex, race)
2. Body weight (e.g., obesity)
3. Physiological and pathological conditions
4. Status of internal organs (e.g., liver, lungs, heart, kidney, stomach, pancreas, bladder)
5. Age (e.g., child, adult, elderly)

Intermediate Factors

1. Substance use (e.g., tobacco, alcohol, drugs)
2. Food and eating habits
3. Stress and mentality

External Factors

1. Climate, ultraviolet light, environmental pollution
2. Quality of medical services, disease diagnosis, care and treatment
3. Patient's compliance
4. Level of education and economy
5. Social and cultural background

Disease onset and progress will be affected by the factors listed above. The onset of disease will be more closely related to personal factors such as daily lifestyle, work, and eating habits. Let's learn some details of each factor and its associated risks to health.

Diet

It is said that one third of cancer cases in the world occur in people living in the US. If we compare the number of cancer occurrences in the rest of the world to the number of cancer occurrences in the US per population, the rate of cancer occurrence in the US will indeed be higher than the rest of the world.

What could be the reason for the higher occurrence of cancer in the US compared to other countries, even though the standard of living for people in the US is better than the rest of the world?

The primary reason for the high incidence of cancer in the US is diet. In terms of cancer risk, a high-calorie diet leading to obesity is as high as the risk of smoking. It should be noted that the larger number of health examinations carried out in the US may contribute to the cancer-incidence numbers, leading to the higher number of cancer incidences reported.

There have been several published scientific articles showing a close relationship between obesity and cancer. Obesity can also negatively impact the prognosis of cancer under treatment. Hence, controlling one's diet to reduce obesity not only helps to prevent the occurrence of cancer, but it can also improve the results of cancer treatment.

Obesity and Cancer

In 2014, the American Society of Clinical Oncology issued their first official statement about obesity and cancer. The announcement stated that although obesity had been known for a long time as the main cause of diabetes and cardiovascular diseases, obesity should now be the core focus in the fight against cancer and the improvement of cancer prognosis.

In November 2014, Dr. Ligibel reported in the *Journal of Clinical Oncology* that it is very important for people to learn about and understand the relationship between obesity and cancer. Obesity accounts for 20% of cancer-related deaths. The risk of obesity-related cancer is as high as tobacco-related cancer.[1]

Over the past 30–40 years, obesity has increased tremendously in the US and other developed countries. Aside from the well-documented finding that obesity causes cardiovascular diseases and diabetes, it is also a critical hidden risk factor in the cause of cancer.

Obesity deteriorates the prognosis of cancer patients who are undergoing long-term treatment and reduces the efficacy of cancer drug treatments. It also increases the risk of co-morbidities and the recurrence of malignant cancer.

The adipose cells in obese patients can push the growth of cancer cells by supporting the production of micro blood vessels around the tumor tissue and providing nutrients for cancer cells.[1]

Reference

1. Jennifer A. Ligibel, MD, Dana-Farber Cancer Institute, *JCO*, November, 2014

Childhood Obesity and Leukemia

In 2014, another important report was issued which related the effect of obesity with leukemia in children. Dr. Mittelman said at the American Association for Cancer Research (AACR) conference that obesity was closely linked to cancer as well as deaths caused by cancer. Further, overweight children have a higher rate of acute leukemia recurrence compared to non-overweight children.[1]

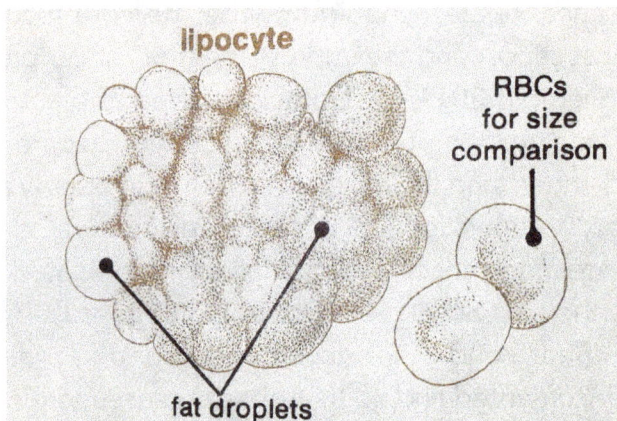

Picture comparing the size of fat droplets to that red blood cells. (From *Mellnoi's Illustrated Medical Dictionary*. The Williams & Wilkins Company.)

Using animal models, one study reported that the survival rate after cancer drug treatment was especially low in obese mice with leukemia. The key points reported in the study include: (i) Adipocytes and fat droplets interfere with and reduce cancer drug absorption into cancer cells; (ii) Adipocytes help cancer cells survive by releasing asparagine, glutamine, fatty acids, and other fuels which facilitate the division and growth of cancer cells; and (iii) Adipocytes interfere with the signal of apoptosis (suicide of cells) in cancer cells.

Doctors sometimes prescribe steroids to young leukemia patients. Such steroid treatments can increase body fat in children by up to 25%. Due to weight gain from the steroid treatment, these children will also have a larger appetite and eat more. This worsens the situation as it decreases the efficacy of drug treatment, thereby reducing the survival rate of young leukemia patients.

According to other studies, the adverse effects of obesity on leukemia patients can be reversed by directly reducing body fat.[2] Dr. Etan Orgel at the Children's Hospital in Los Angeles reported that the efficacy of anti-cancer drug treatments for patients with reduced obesity was higher compared to similar treatments for obese patients.[3]

In conclusion, obesity is significantly related to cancer as a direct cause of cancer as well as a worsening factor in the prognosis of cancer patients. Thus, the control of obesity is important not only for the general maintenance of health but also for cancer patients undergoing treatment.

References

1. Mittelman SD. Childhood obesity and leukemia: Opportunities for intervention. *AACR* International Conference on Frontiers in Cancer Prevention Research. September 30, 2014.
2. Calle EE, Rodriguez C, Walker-Thurmond K, *et al.* Overweight, obesity, and mortality from cancer in a prospectively studied cohort of U.S. adults. *N Engl J Med* **348**:1625–1638, 2003.
3. Orgel E, Sposto R, Malvar J, *et al.* Impact on survival and toxicity by duration of weight extremes during treatment for pediatric acute lymphoblastic leukemia. *J Clin Oncol* **32**:1331–1337, 2014.

Prevention of Breast Cancer should Start from Age Two

Dr. Graham A. Colditz, from the Institute for Public Health at Washington University in St. Louis, recommended that preventive steps against breast cancer should start from as early as age two. As old habits die hard, good habits should be cultivated from a young age to help prevent the disease.

Good habits that formed in early childhood can create the foundations needed to reduce the occurrence of breast cancer by up to 70%. Conversely, changing habits in mid-adulthood to prevent breast cancer is estimated to have only a 50% reduction rate.

The growth of breast cells and tissues is very active and fast during the time between a female's first menstruation and the birth of her first baby. If a woman develops bad habits such as eating high-calorie foods including large amounts of animal proteins and alcohol drinking while lacking physical exercise, she will have an elevated risk of getting breast cancer.

Maintaining a healthy lifestyle and cultivating good eating habits from early childhood is strongly recommended to avoid the occurrence of breast cancer.

Smoking

Severe health problems caused by smoking or indirect smoking are already well known, but many people still pick up and persist in smoking. Millions of people suffer from many complex diseases caused by smoking. Smoking-related health issues are not only limited to respiratory problems but also include other aspects of the body. Diseases caused by or related to smoking include emphysema of the lung, chronic obstructive pulmonary disease

(COPD), lung cancer, diabetes, high blood pressure, stroke, heart attack, and cancers in various other organs and tissues.

According to a report in October 2014, 14 million new patients are diagnosed with health problems every year in the United States due to smoking. Among these patients, 7.5 million suffer from shortness of breath due to COPD.

A study published in the *Journal of the American Medical Association: Internal Medicine* listed the top four major diseases caused by smoking as[1]:

- Heart attack: 2.3 million cases
- Cancer: 1.3 million cases
- Stroke: 1.2 million cases
- Diabetes: 1.8 million cases

Reference

1. *JAMA* Internal Medicine October 13, 2014.

Key Points — To Avoid Exposure to Potential Toxic Substances in Everyday Life

As explained in the earlier chapters of this book, toxicological risk is based on the conditions of exposure to toxic substances. To reduce toxicological risk, we should try not to expose ourselves to toxic chemical substances in our daily lives. The following five points should be remembered and practiced as much as possible in order to maintain a healthy lifestyle with reduced toxicity.

1. Living conditions: choose residential areas with fresh air, clean water, and nature (e.g., forests, parks) rather than residential areas with smog, dust, and polluted water.

2. Eating habits: form good eating habits as early as possible, consume more natural foods, and avoid a diet that is high in calories or processed with various artificial ingredients.

3. Lifestyle practices: try not to use products containing ingredients such as antibacterial agents, excessive amount of fragrances, and volatile organic compounds. Consumers should be aware of potential harmful substances in products before buying and using them.

4. Exposure to recreational carcinogens: cut down on or avoid cigarette smoking, excessive alcohol drinking, and narcotic drugs.

5. Exercise habits: improve the immune system with exercise.

It is estimated that up to 50% of cancer cases and deaths can be prevented if people upkeep simple, healthy lifestyles including healthy eating, regular physical activity, and reduced tobacco and alcohol consumption alongside cancer prevention activities such as cancer screenings and vaccinations.

Start of Cancer and Patients' Ordeal

What is DNA?

Deoxyribonucleic acid (DNA) is a double helix formed by base pairs attached to a sugar-phosphate backbone. DNA is comprised of four chemical bases: adenine (A), cytosine (C), guanine (G), and thymine (T). These nucleobases weave together into a nucleic acid chain, forming a twisted spiral ladder called the double helix. The sequence of the bases A, C, G, and T determines the information available for building and maintaining an organism.

An important property of DNA is that it can replicate or, in other words, make copies of itself. Each strand of DNA in the double helix can serve as a pattern for duplicating the sequence of bases. This is critical when cells divide as each new cell needs to have an exact copy of the DNA present in the old cell.

A gene is a sequence of DNA. During gene expression, the DNA is first copied into ribonucleic acid (RNA). The RNA can be directly functional or serve as an intermediate template for a protein that performs a function. About 95% of the DNA

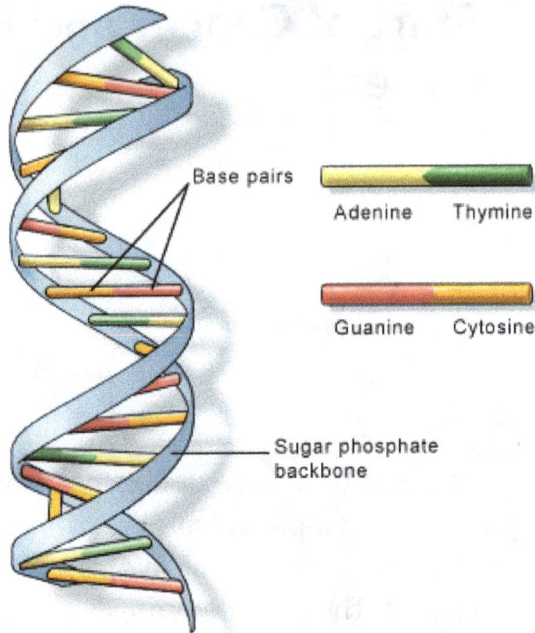

Base pairs

Adenine   Thymine

Guanine   Cytosine

Sugar phosphate
backbone

U.S. National Library of Medicine

Credit: US National Library of Medicine.

are inactive; only the rest of the 5% of DNA, consisting of more than 100,000 individual genes, are actively involved in making proteins. Each gene works to synthesize proteins with appropriate combinations of A, C, G, and T nucleotide bases, according to the genetic information in it.

Gene mutations can occur from external stress factors that interfere with the integrity of the nucleotide base sequences. Gene mutations lead to erroneous combinations of A, C, G, and T nucleobases, producing abnormal proteins that do not function appropriately which can eventually cause diseases like cancer.

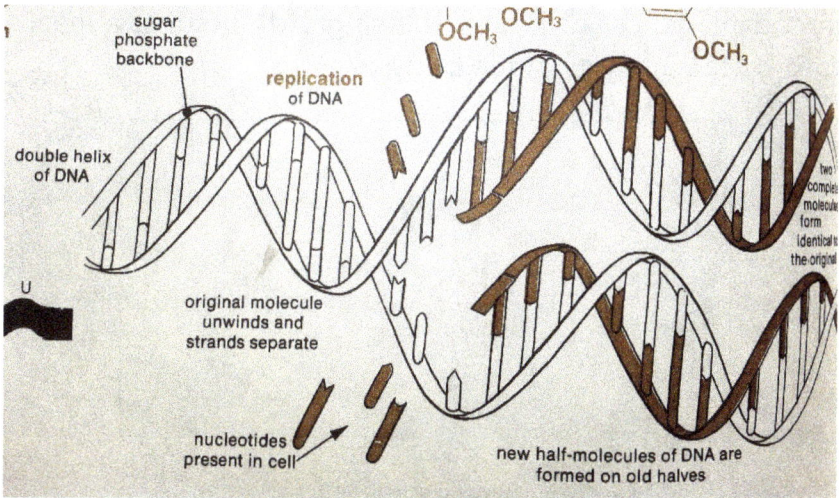

DNA replication during cell division.

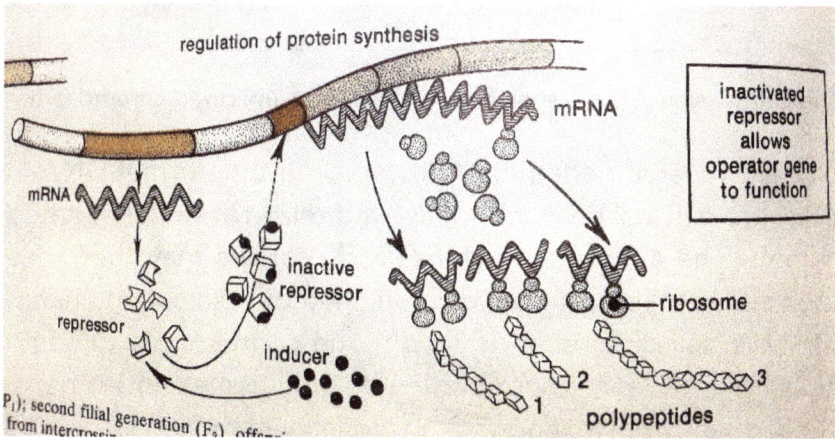

Protein synthesis carried out by gene and messenger RNA.

Fundamental Cause of Cancer

Division and growth of cells in humans occur only when necessary. That is, only when the body is in need of growth or repair from damage, cell division and their growth occur as a means to keep the integrity of the body.

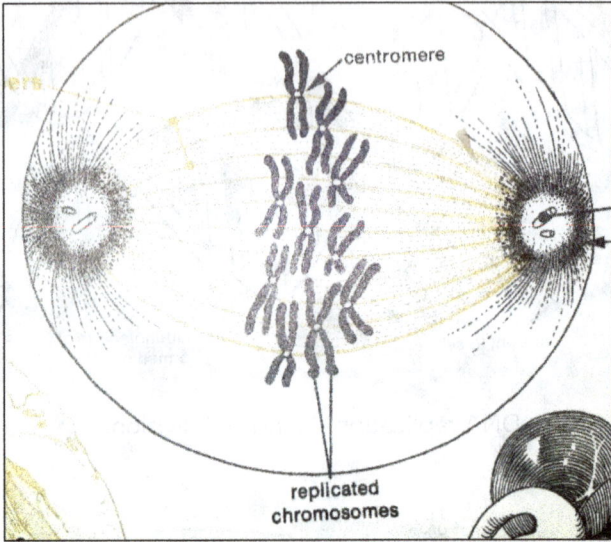

The cell division process showing the division of replicated chromosomes.

However, if gene mutations occur in the normal DNA in cells, proteins will be inaccurately synthesized from the mutated signals. The abnormally synthesized proteins may then lose their ability to regulate cell division, thereby resulting in uncontrollable cell division and growth. The continuously dividing cells will invade into surrounding healthy tissues and organs, subsequently destroying the functionality of those tissues and organs. This is the disease that we call cancer.

Contrary to other diseases, cancer does not result from an invasion of external cancer cells into the human body. Instead, cancer arises internally from uncontrollable cell division as a result of gene mutations.

Gene mutations are caused by external carcinogenic factors such as smoking, alcohol drinking, industrial pollutants, bacteria, viruses, ultraviolet light, radiation, unhealthy eating, and various other toxic substances that people are exposed to in daily life. (Refer to Chapters 1–3 for details of potential toxic substances in daily life, and how these toxic substances react in the body, leading to disease.)

Although gene mutations may occur in the body, these mutations can be reversed or repaired if the body's immune system is strong and functional. An effective immune system can identify and destroy cells with gene mutations, thereby preventing the onset of cancer. However, when the immune system is weak, it will be unable to repair or reverse gene mutations, leaving the body vulnerable to cancer.

Cancer Prevention

The ultimate way to avoid cancer is to prevent normal cells from being affected by gene or DNA mutations. When normal genes mutate into abnormal genes in the cells, the normal cells can turn cancerous.

Another way to prevent cancer is to repair the genetic mutations that have already occurred in our cells or to remove cells that have been damaged from our body. This protective way of cancer prevention already exists in us, though we cannot see it. There is no perfect way to avoid cancer in our lifetime. However, the probability of getting cancer can be minimized if people try to minimize exposure to toxic chemical substances in daily life while they keep their strong immune system in the body by doing regular exercise and maintaining a healthy diet.

In summary, cancer is avoidable by (i) minimizing exposure to pollutants and toxic substances in daily life, and (ii) keeping a strong immunity in the body with regular exercise and healthy eating habits.

Agony of Cancer Patients and the Difficulties they have to Deal with

Patients who are diagnosed with cancer typically become gripped with fear and stress due to their lack of knowledge regarding the disease. When patients meet doctors at the hospital, they feel helpless and desperate for guidance because they do not know much about the disease. Most cancer patients simply follow the directions given by their doctor without a sufficient understanding of their disease condition, such as the type and stage of cancer, available treatment plans, post-treatment options, risks and benefits associated with each type of treatment, quality of life, economic burden, probability of cancer recurrence, supportive care, and passage towards the end of life.

In many big hospitals or cancer centers around the world, doctors often do not have enough time to explain comprehensively to patients about the cancer treatment process and the options available. Moreover, even if doctors had sufficient time to explain the details, many patients will still be unable to fully appreciate the information if they do not have a basic knowledge of the disease.

As medical doctors are specially trained to tackle the disease, it is essential that patients follow and comply with their doctors' advice. In addition, it is highly recommended that patients learn as much as possible about the cancer they have been diagnosed with, as well as the corresponding treatment options and long-term coping strategies if patients want to get better outcomes from treatments. Patients and doctors should work together as a team to address the disease. Educated patients are likely to have a better understanding of their disease and treatment options. Thus, they can work more effectively with their doctors.

Here is an example of a sad case encountered by an Asian patient who died in early 2014. The 56 year-old patient had lost 25 kg in five months. Later, he was diagnosed with a rare disease — called β amyloidosis — but no appropriate drug was available at that time to treat the disease. Doctors recommended the use of chemotherapy and steroids even though the patient did not have cancer. The patient received one cycle of chemotherapy as recommended; however, he died within two months after the treatment.

On hindsight, would it have been better if the patient was not treated with chemotherapy? From a toxicological viewpoint, he should not have attempted to treat his disease using the highly toxic anti-cancer drug since he was already in a state that was too weak to tolerate the chemotherapy.

Was there any good rationale to administer the anti-cancer treatment to this patient who was already weakened with a rare and non-cancerous disease, even if the anti-cancer drug was not the right one to use?

The Minds of Patients and Doctors

As medical service providers, doctors may feel that they are caring for the patient by recommending more tests for patients to do. At the same time, patients also feel like they are being cared for as they go through these tests.

Most patients desperately want to be cured. It is human nature that patients are willing to try any possible medical treatments in hopes of curing their disease. Therefore, it is often difficult for doctors to say no to patients when they are desperate to try anything for their life. At the same time, doctors may also be curious to know if a particular new drug might work and be tempted to test the new drug on eager patients.

When people get sick with a difficult disease, they tend to plunge into an unstable situation both physically and psychologically. This desperate and difficult situation compels them to seek any help so that they can get cured.

Excessive Medical Services

The mission of hospitals and doctors is to cure patients of their illnesses. With their medical knowledge and the medical tools available from the health industry, doctors help to advise and treat patients. The goal is to use the best possible medicines or medical devices to treat patients and to cure them.

In a sense, doctors, hospitals, and pharmaceutical companies are partners in the endeavor to provide patients with quality medical services. A positive aspect of the partnership between pharmaceutical companies and doctors/hospitals is that patients can get the best medical services available. On the other hand, this partnership can sometimes lead to excessive medical treatment for patients. Excessive medical treatment may unnecessarily increase the medical expenses of patients while worsening the quality of life of late-stage cancer patients.

What Should I do if I have Cancer?

Do not worry too much if you get diagnosed with cancer. Nowadays, cancer no longer equates to a death sentence. In principle, a life with cancer is not very different from a life with other types of disease.

The onset of cancer begins from DNA/gene mutations when a person's immune protection system is not working well. After the onset of cancer, if a patient can maintain a strong immune system, the cancer can be resolved and the patient will be able to prolong his or her life.

Just like other diseases, some patients may get cured, some may live with the cancer for many more years, and some may face an early death, depending on the status of their immune system and health condition.

By taking advantage of current anti-cancer treatment options and innovative new drugs under development, if cancer patients can maintain a good immune system, keeping their body strong, they will be able to survive for many years or even have more chances of getting cured. With the advance of medical technology and innovative cancer drug development, cancer may be classified as a common curable disease like a flu in the future. Thus don't panic when you are diagnosed with cancer, and study your cancer and related treatment options available with a positive mindset.

Most importantly, do not panic if you are diagnosed with cancer.

Chapter 5

Types of Cancer

To help readers get a better understanding of the types, categories, and classifications of cancer, it will be useful to introduce some of the common scientific jargon associated with the disease.

Cancer is categorized mainly according to the main organ in which it originated as well as its type of organization and tissue. Next, it will be further classified into stages and grades according to the evaluation systems describing the extent of cancer. The most appropriate treatment options will then be decided based on the cancer type identified and its classifications.

To confirm the cancer type and its classifications, patients may undergo radiological examinations such as computed tomography (CT) scans, magnetic resonance imaging (MRI), positron emission tomography (PET) scans, pathology tests or even gene mutation tests.

Staging of Cancer

Prior to commencing any cancer treatment, it is necessary to find out how far the cancer has spread or what "stage" it has reached. Staging is a system that is used to classify the extent

Resources: American Joint Committee on Cancer, www.cancerstaging.org

of cancer and to decide which treatment options would be ideal for patients.

Usually, the doctor will estimate the stage of cancer at the time of diagnosis and do further tests to confirm the "clinical stage" of the disease. A pathologist will examine the tumor tissue and assign the cancer a "pathologic stage." In general, the pathologic stage is the most important piece of information in deciding the treatment approach.

What is the TNM System?

Doctors, physicians, and scientists use the standard tumor, lymph node, and metastasis (TNM) system to do staging for most cancers. The TNM system was developed and continually updated by the American Joint Committee on Cancer.

The most common cancers that doctors stage using the TNM system are breast, colon, renal, stomach, esophagus, pancreas, and lung cancers. Other cancers that are staged with the TNM system include soft tissue sarcoma and melanoma. Staging systems exist for 52 sites or types of cancer.

Some cancers are not staged using the TNM system, such as cancers of the blood, bone marrow, and the brain. Gynecologic cancers use another staging system which doctors can translate into TNM.

TNM Staging

- T (Tumor): tumor size, extent, or penetration.
- N (Nodes): the number of lymph nodes with cancer or the location of the cancer-involved lymph nodes.

- M (Metastasis): distant metastasis or the spread of the cancer to other parts of the body, which indicates whether there are cancer cells outside the local area of the tumor and its surrounding lymph nodes.

  T: size or direct extent of the primary tumor

- Tx: tumor cannot be evaluated
- Tis: carcinoma *in situ*, which refers to a group of abnormal cells or pre-cancer cells
- T0: no signs of tumor
- T1, T2, T3, or T4: size and/or extent of the primary tumor, classified according to size and involvement in surrounding tissues

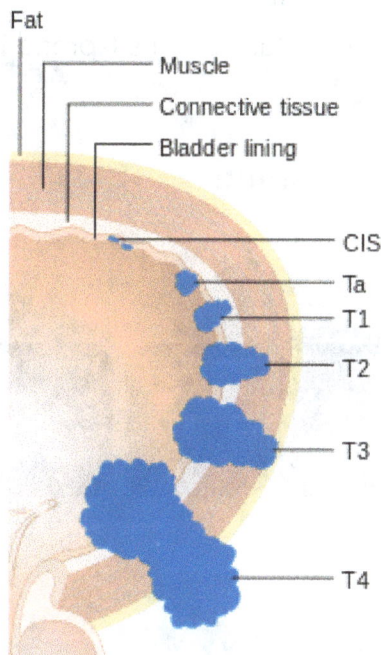

Diagram showing the T stages of bladder cancer.

N: degree of spread to regional lymph nodes

- Nx: lymph nodes cannot be evaluated
- N0: tumor cells absent in regional lymph nodes
- N1: tumor cells present in regional lymph nodes (at some sites: tumor spread to closest or small number of regional lymph nodes)
- N2: tumor spread to an extent between N1 and N3 (N2 is not used at all sites)
- N3: tumor spread to more distant or numerous regional lymph nodes (N3 is not used at all sites)

M: presence of distant metastasis

- M0: no distant metastasis
- M1: metastasis to distant organs (spread beyond regional lymph nodes)

Overall Stage Grouping

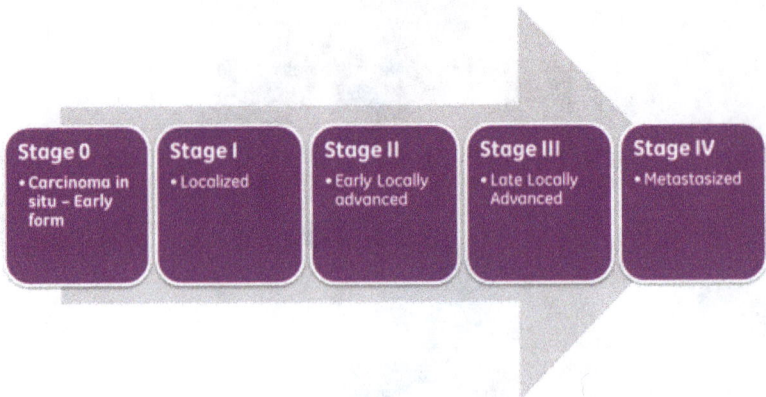

Stage 0	Stage I	Stage II	Stage III	Stage IV
• Carcinoma in situ – Early form	• Localized	• Early Locally advanced	• Late Locally Advanced	• Metastasized

Overall Stage Grouping is referred to as Roman Numeral Staging to describe the progression of cancer.

- **Stage 0:** carcinoma *in situ*; the cancer is confined to the epidermal cells only.
- **Stage I:** cancers are localized to one part of the body; the original tumor is small and confined within the organ it started in.

  → *Stage I cancer can be surgically removed if small enough.*
- **Stage II:** cancers are locally advanced and have spread to lymph nodes close to the tumor.

  → *Stage II cancer can be treated by chemotherapy, radiation, or surgery.*
- **Stage III:** cancers are locally advanced and have spread to lymph nodes and surrounding tissues; the specific criteria for Stages II and III differ according to diagnosis.

  → *Stage III cancer can be treated by chemotherapy, radiation, or surgery.*
- **Stage IV:** cancers have metastasized and spread to other organs or throughout the body.

  → *Stage IV cancer can be treated by chemotherapy, radiation, or surgery.*

What does "Stage Grouping" Mean?

Once doctors have determined the TNM categories, they can classify the cancer into a "stage group." Stage grouping uses Roman numerals I, II, III, or IV, with a larger number representing a more advanced stage of cancer.

If a patient takes a part in a clinical trial to assess his or her cancer, the stage group of the cancer must be known first as it will allow the patient to be placed into an appropriate treatment group. (A clinical trial is a research study that is conducted, with the patient's permission, to investigate how effective and safe a new drug treatment is.)

Staging is a system that allows doctors and practitioners to classify the extent of cancer and to decide what treatment options would work best for their patients.

Grades of Cancer Cells

Grading in cancer is different from staging. While staging is a measure of the extent to which the cancer has spread, grading is a measure of the cell appearance in tumors.

The cancer grade is a description of how abnormal the cancer cells appear when compared to surrounding normal tissue. The grades are given from 1 to 4.

- Grade 1: well-differentiated cells that look relatively similar to surrounding normal cells with only slightly unusual forms of separation (*low grade → slow growing cells*)
- Grade 2: moderately differentiated cells with more unusual forms compared to Grade 1 (*intermediate grade*)
- Grade 3: poorly differentiated cells with unusual forms; cancer cells look abnormal and lack normal tissue structure (*high grade → grow rapidly and spread fast*)
- Grade 4: undifferentiated cells; cancer cells are immature and cannot be distinguished from primitive forms (*high grade → grow rapidly and spread fast*)

Types of Cancer Based on the Origin of Organs or Tissues

1. Carcinoma
2. Sarcoma
3. Myeloma
4. Leukemia
5. Lymphoma
6. Mixed Types

Carcinoma

Carcinoma is a type of cancer that develops from epithelial cells or within tissues that line the inner or outer surfaces of the body. This cancer accounts for 80% to 90% of all cancers.

Sarcoma

Sarcoma are malignant tumors made of cancellous bone, cartilage, fat, muscle, vascular, or hematopoietic tissues.

Myeloma

Known as multiple myeloma or plasma cell myeloma, myeloma is a cancer of plasma cells, a type of white blood cells that are normally responsible for producing antibodies.

Leukemia

Leukemia is a group of cancers that usually begins in the bone marrow and eventually manifests as a high number of abnormal white blood cells. These white blood cells are not fully developed and are called blasts or leukemia cells. Leukemia can be further broken down into the following.

- *Myelogenous* or *granulocytic leukemia*: cancerous change that takes place in the marrow cells responsible for forming red blood cells, some white blood cells, and platelets.
- *Lymphoblastic leukemia*: cancerous change that takes place in a particular type of marrow cells responsible for forming lymphocytes, which are infection-fighting immune system cells.
- *Polycythemia vera* or *erythremia*: bone marrow disease that leads to an abnormal increase in the number of blood cells, especially red blood cells.

Cell Type	Acute	Chronic
Lymphocytic leukemia (or "lymphoblastic")	Acute lymphoblastic leukemia	Chronic lympho- cytic leukemia
Myelogenous leukemia ("myeloid" or "non-lymphocytic")	Acute myelogenous leu- kemia (or myeloblastic)	Chronic myeloge- nous leukemia

Lymphoma

Lymphoma is a cancer that originates in the immune system's infection-fighting cells, also known as lymphocytes. These cells are found in the lymph nodes, spleen, tonsils, thymus, and other parts of the body. Lymphoma is different from leukemia — lymphoma starts in infection-fighting cells whereas leukemia starts from blood-forming cells inside the bone marrow.

The two main categories of lymphoma are (1) Hodgkin's lymphoma and (2) non-Hodgkin's lymphoma. Hodgkin's lymphoma is marked by the presence of a type of cells called the Reed-Sternberg cells, while all other lymphomas are catego- rized as non-Hodgkin's lymphomas.

Mixed types

Mixed types of cancers originate from a variety of tissues or organs. Some examples include:

- Adenosquamous carcinoma
- Mixed mesodermal tumor
- Carcinosarcoma
- Teratocarcinoma

Classification by the Main Organ where the Cancer Originated

Cancer is typically classified according to the organ it started in. Examples include lung cancer, stomach cancer, colorectal cancer, pancreatic cancer, liver cancer, brain cancer, head and neck cancer, oral cancer, skin cancer, kidney cancer, bladder cancer, prostate cancer, breast cancer, and ovarian cancer.

Which Category or Classification does my Cancer Belong to? What Kinds of Genetic Mutations Occurred in the Formation of my Cancer?

We have learnt that there are various types of cancer and they are categorized according to the organ or tissue of origin. We have also learnt that cancer is classified into stages and grades according to the TNM staging system and the pathological grading of cancer cells respectively.

To accurately evaluate the stage and grade of cancers, doctors use scanning and imaging tools. Nowadays, doctors can also conduct tests to determine the specific gene mutations that caused the cancer, such as HER2, RAS, BRAF, KRAS, EGFR, ALK, and p53, etc., though the technology of gene mutation test is rapidly evolving but it is not feasible yet to cover all cancer types at this moment.

These forms of modern technology are useful in helping us evaluate the extent of cancer and enabling us to choose the best treatment options, such as surgery, chemotherapy, radiotherapy, or a combination of treatment, target therapy, and immunotherapy.

Chapter

6

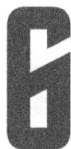

Understanding Anti-Cancer Drugs and Treatment

Chemotherapy

Chemotherapy is the administering of toxins that attack the microtubules or other molecules of cancer cells, resulting in the death of cancer cells or stopping their growth. However, massive non-targeted attacks can also cause collateral damage to normal cells in the body, thereby causing toxic side effects.

For example, Paclitaxel (commercially named Taxol), a bioactive compound extracted from yew trees, has been a prime non-target chemotherapy drug in the market for decades. The drug is intravenously administered in weekly, bi-weekly, or tri-weekly treatment cycles at various doses. The number of cycles can be short or long depending on the patient's response to the drug.

Usually, upon receiving cycles of chemotherapy, the size of the tumor will be reduced. On rare occasions, tumors may disappear post-treatment. However, most patients experience the recurrence of tumors in a few months or years after the completion of chemotherapy.

The weakness of traditional chemotherapy is that side effects can be very severe. Common side effects from chemo-therapy include hair loss, diarrhea, decreased white blood cells, neuropathy, anorexia, hand-foot syndrome, depression, high blood pressure, abdominal pain, vomiting, muscular pain, and neuralgia.

Radiotherapy

Traditionally, radiotherapy is used together with chemotherapy. Like chemotherapy, radiotherapy also has adverse side effects. Radiotherapy can be administered before or after surgery, or during the course of cancer treatment.

Target Drug Therapy

As a form of chemotherapy, target drug therapy specifically attacks cancer cells by binding to specific receptors or molecules on cancer cells and inhibiting their vital functions.

Genetic mutation tests before starting treatment with a target anti-cancer drug — Unlike normal cells, cancer cells may present some unique characteristics that can be exploited to identify and specifically attack them. Therefore, before target anti-cancer drugs are administered to patients, the hospital will carry out molecular biology tests that can check for the presence of specific target receptors that the anti-cancer drugs can bind to. In other words, based on the genetic test results, appropriate anti-cancer drugs that are capable of homing in specifically on those target receptors will be administered to patients with the relevant gene mutations, resulting in more effective and personalized anti-cancer treatment.

For example, some breast cancer cells have 100 times more HER2 receptors on their cell walls compared to normal cells. Thus, a monoclonal antibody drug with a HER2 antigen that binds to the extracellular HER2 domain of cancer cells can aid the body's immune system in specifically stunting the proliferation of breast cancer cells.

Inhibiting the creation of new blood vessels by cancer cells — Cancer cells make their own blood vessels by forming a microcirculation environment to acquire nutrients and oxygen for survival and growth. A target drug like Axitinib inhibits the cancer cells' creation of new blood vessels by selectively binding to the VEGF receptors 1, 2, and 3 on target cancer cells, thus preventing new blood vessels from forming and inhibiting the growth of cancer.

Anti-angiogenesis drug — There are several target drug therapies that exhibit anti-angiogenesis effects on cancer cells. These drugs target specific molecules on the cancer cells. After the drug binds to or blocks specific molecules on the cancer cells, the generation of micro-blood vessels is inhibited or retarded. The pictures below show the effects of anti-angiogenesis drugs on the formation of micro-blood vessels.

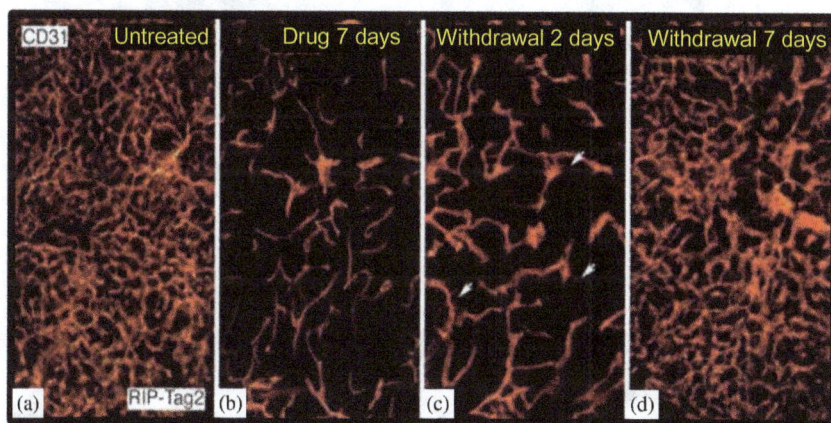

Image courtesy of Pfizer Inc.

a. Blood vessels aggressively forming in the tumor tissue
b. Blood vessels significantly reduced after 7 days of drug treatment
c. Blood vessels re-forming two days after drug treatment has stopped
d. Blood vessels proliferating again 7 days after drug treatment has stopped

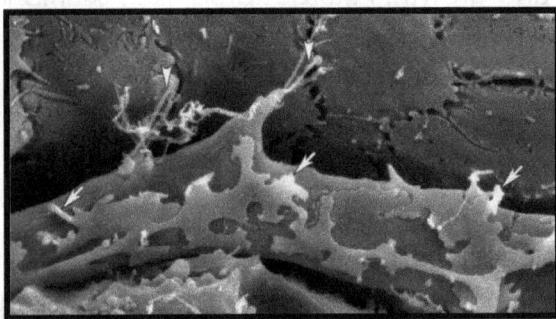

Formation of micro-blood vessels in tumor tissue.

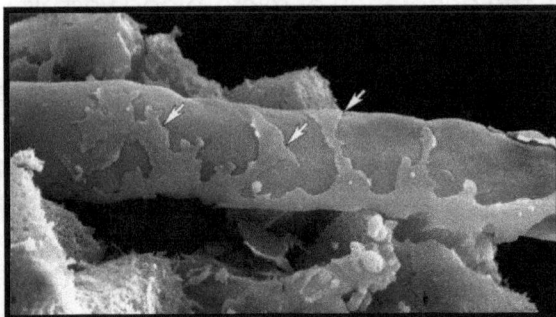

Inhibition of the formation of micro-blood vessels formation in tumor tissue after 7 days of drug treatment.

Benefits of target drug therapy — Target anti-cancer drugs aim specifically at receptors or molecules on cancer cells. In other words, target anti-cancer drugs block the activity of the specific receptors on cancer cells, thereby inhibiting their growth and spread. As target anti-cancer drugs work specifically against cancer cells, they have better anti-cancer efficacy compared to traditional non-specific chemotherapy.

Limits of target drug therapy — When cancer cells are attacked by any type of anti-cancer drugs, the cancer cells will try to survive by either modifying their specific gene receptors or finding ways to neutralize the drug. Once cancer cells find new means of survival from these anti-cancer drugs, they will be able to sustain themselves and grow and spread again.

Although target anti-cancer drugs have less side effects compared to traditional chemotherapy, some side effects may still arise as target anti-cancer drugs can also bind to similar target molecules in non-cancerous cells. Thus, these normal cells may also be affected when the target anti-cancer drugs are used.

Side effects from target anti-cancer drugs vary depending on the type of drugs used. Common side effects that have been reported include diarrhea, high blood pressure, hand-foot syndrome, skin disease, skin dryness, itchiness, hair change, body hair growth, and changes in thyroid hormone levels.

Antibody-drug Conjugates — Monoclonal Antibodies Combined with Chemical Drugs

Antibody-drug conjugates (ADCs) are made by combining monoclonal antibodies and cytotoxic drugs. As antibodies have the unique ability to seek out cancer cells, they can target cancer cells and bind them with the combined cytotoxic drug. When ADC is administered to patients, it works like a homing missile — the ADC is locked in to the cancer cells and the cytotoxic drug destroys them. Animal studies and human clinical trials with ADCs look very promising.

Drug-induced Cell Suicide (Apoptosis)

When normal cells are attacked by viruses and bacteria, the cells get irreversibly damaged at the cellular DNA level. The permanently damaged cells will then commit suicide according to biological signals from the body, a process that is known as apoptosis. By committing suicide and dismantling themselves from the body, they protect neighboring healthy cells and tissues from further infection, thereby maintaining the health of the rest of the body.

The tumor suppressor gene, p53, is switched on in abnormal cells. Switching on p53 gene in abnormal cells is an intracellular signal to get the cells to commit suicide. The suicided cells are subsequently destroyed by caspases and removed by the body's immune cells.

However, if p53 gene is mutated and cannot function properly in abnormal cells to induce the signal for apoptosis, the abnormal cells will divide continuously. An example is the human papilloma virus (HPV), which interferes with p53 gene's signaling ability in cervical cancer patients. This interference prevents cells from committing suicide and causes these cells to divide continuously, thereby leading to cancer.

Many research and development activities are currently ongoing with p53 gene. The aim is to develop new and effective target anti-cancer drugs through a better understanding of p53 gene's ability to induce apoptosis as well as HPV's interference with the apoptosis signal.

Immune Therapy

If cancer cells appear within the body, the body will launch its own immune cells to fight them. However, cancer cells can exploit the checkpoint inhibitor proteins known as the programmed cell death protein (PD-1) and its ligand (PD-L1) to neutralize the attack of immune cells. When immune cells are neutralized, the cancer cells can survive and proliferate.

PD-1 acts like a brake on the immune system, preventing the activation of natural killer cells known as T-cells. Cancer cells can make PD-L1 proteins that bind to the PD-1 protein and block the activation of immune cells. By doing so, cancer cells can curb attacks from immune cells and continue to survive and grow. Newly developed immune therapy drugs work to release the brakes put in place by PD-1 and induce the activation of immune cells to attack cancer cells.

New immune therapy drugs do not attack cancer cells directly but instead utilize the mechanism of PD-1 and PD-L1 proteins to reactivate our immune cells that are naturally designed to fight cancer cells. While clinical studies of this innovative therapy look promising, it does not work for all types of cancer or for all patients and has been documented to have some undesirable side effects. More studies are ongoing with these new forms of immunotherapy drugs.

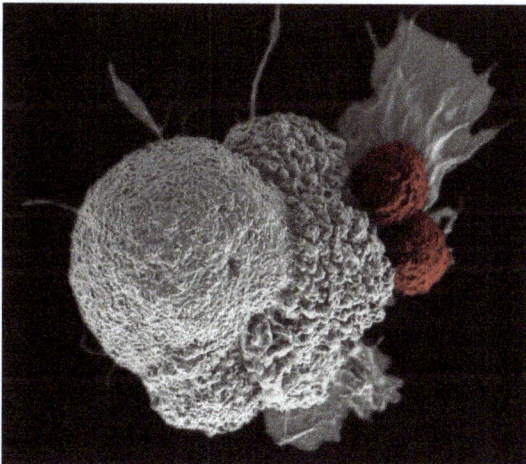

Cancer immunotherapy in action: An oral cancer cell (white) is attacked by two T cells (red) as part of the body's immune response. (Rita Elena Serda/Duncan Comprehensive Cancer Center at Baylor College of Medicine via NCI.)

Next-Generation Virus Vaccines

Currently, HPV vaccines are being widely administered to young women for the prevention of cervical cancer. HPV vaccines are recommended for young men as well. This antivirus vaccine is aimed at preventing the occurrence of the cancer rather than treating it after it has already occurred.

Antivirus therapy may be another effective way to fight cancer in future. An interesting report was published in 2014 regarding a woman from Minnesota who was over 50 years of age and suffered from end-stage bone marrow cancer. After experiencing failures in chemotherapy and stem cell transplants, she was treated with very high doses of measles vaccine as a last resort. Surprisingly, all the cancer cells were destroyed within three days of the treatment and the patient got cured. In this fluke attempt, the measles vaccine killed only the cancer cells while leaving the patient's normal cells untouched.

To confirm the effectiveness of such antivirus therapies, more studies will be needed with larger numbers of patients using the vaccine. This lone successful case will be a cornerstone for developing re-engineered antivirus therapy drugs for cancer patients.

Reference

1.   Mayo Clinic Proceedings, May 2014.

7 Chemotherapy and the Management of Quality of Life

Surgery and Chemotherapy

Unlike blood cancers, solid tumor cancers usually require surgery and chemotherapy. Sometimes, chemotherapy is used before surgery to help shrink the size of cancer lumps. Of course, the main reason for surgery is to remove at least a major chunk of the tumor, if not the entire tumor.

Early stage tumors, as a form of non-invasive cancer, are typically small and in situ (in its place). Therefore, it is easy to remove early stage tumors from the surrounding tissue. As tumors reach the mid or later stage, however, the tumor mass becomes larger or more invasive in neighboring tissues, thus becoming harder to remove.

CT, MRI, and PET scans are a great help in guiding the surgical removal of tumors from the body. However, current imaging technologies have a limitation — they cannot show all the cancer cells at a micro level in the body, making it difficult to completely remove all cancers from the body.

When cancer patients undergo "successful" surgeries, this means that the tumor mass, at a macro level, was removed while undetected micro-level cancer cells remain. Therefore, following the surgery, patients will need to go for a few cycles of chemotherapy to kill off the remaining cancer cells or inhibit their growth.

In the case of late-stage cancer, cancer cells in the body are usually transmitted or metastasized to other tissues or organs. In this case, the doctor may perform either surgery to remove the major tumor mass or chemotherapy without surgery.

Coping with Side Effects from Anti-Cancer Medication

Painful side effects from chemotherapy — how should patients cope?

Patients often face very painful side effects from several cycles of chemotherapy. A case study reported that one third of breast cancer patients have considered committing suicide due to the deterioration of quality of life during chemotherapy treatment. However, if we equip ourselves with sufficient knowledge on chemotherapy treatments, their side effects, and how to cope with them, then the journey ahead will not be so difficult.

Chemotherapy is targeted at killing cancer cells that are rapidly dividing. However, chemotherapy drugs also attack fast-growing normal cells or cells undergoing cell division in our body (e.g., body hair, white blood cells, nails, gastrointestinal epithelial cells, skin, immune cells, etc). Thus, patients treated with chemotherapy often experience severe side effects and toxicity during the treatment. These grueling side effects from chemotherapy can cause some patients to lose the motivation to fight on with life and think of letting it go.

However, it is highly possible for patients to overcome the difficulties of side effects. First, patients should follow the instructions given by the hospital to manage the side effects from the treatment. Next, patients should try to get a positive mindset, maintain his or her own physical strength and immunity to get through the treatment period, and work towards completing the treatment. Then, after completion of chemotherapy, full recovery in a few weeks or months is highly possible.

Here is a good example to share. A Singaporean woman in her late 30s was diagnosed with early-stage breast cancer. She underwent surgery followed by four cycles of chemotherapy using a cocktail of three anti-cancer drugs, namely Herceptin, Taxotere, and Cyclophosphamide. As expected, side effects followed alongside the chemotherapy. Hair loss was a short-term side effect and it only lasted during the duration of chemotherapy. With her hair gone, the patient started putting on hair wigs, hats, and bandanas as her new fashion statement. Three months after the last dose of chemotherapy, her hair started re-growing. Within a year, a full length of hair was present again. "I think more than anything, a woman would be worried about hair loss as a side effect, but there was no physical pain during the hair loss process. There were much more painful and near-death side-effects that I had experienced such as high fever due to febrile neutropenia, diarrhea, allergic skin rash, and anaphylaxis, which were more difficult to endure," she said.

Now in her mid-40s, the patient is completely recovered and back to normal. She is in good health, doing well at work, and having a good family life. She returns to the hospital only for routine checkups.

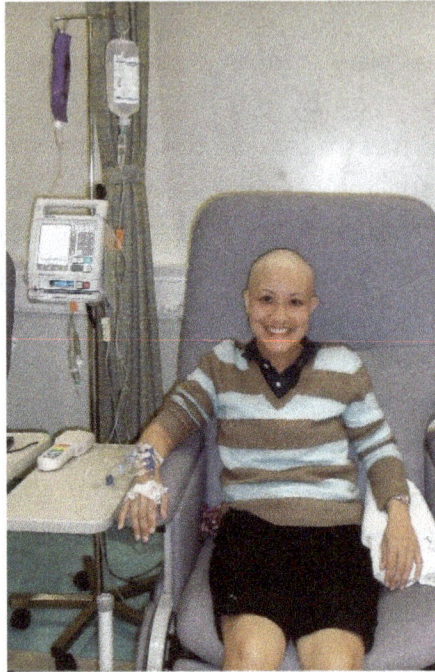

A cancer survivor who overcame chemotherapy positively and completely returned to normal life.

Gain Information about the Side Effects of Anti-Cancer Drugs

Doctors will prescribe medicines to help suppress the side effects that are known to come with anti-cancer drugs. In addition, doctors will provide information about these side effects to allow patients to be prepared and cope with side effects effectively.

The patient may take the coping medication before or after the experience of side effects. Some side effects can be anticipated and proactively treated. For example, several anti-cancer drugs can cause skin-related side effects. If patients knew this information in advance, they can look out for signs such as patchy skin to detect the onset of side effects, thereby getting treatment early and reducing the severity of these side effects. Patients are therefore encouraged to learn about the anticipated side effects from chemotherapy and communicate closely with their doctor to proactively manage the side effects.

Acupuncture Alleviates Symptoms Associated with Cancer Care

Acupuncture is the stimulation of specific points on the body via the insertion of thin metal needles through the skin. Acupuncture has been widely practiced for thousands of years in Asian countries as a traditional medical tool to treat various types of symptoms in people.

Many clinical studies have found that acupuncture can help with certain pains such as back pain, knee pain, headaches, and osteoarthritis with few side effects.[1]

Extensive investigations of the therapeutic modality of acupuncture in Western medical settings have confirmed its efficacy in the clinical management of pain and other symptoms. In oncological settings, research has also demonstrated that acupuncture can significantly reduce symptoms associated with cancer and cancer treatments. This modality has proven to be very safe; serious adverse effects are rare or nonexistent among randomized controlled trials.[2]

The most solid supporting evidence in oncology comes from studies of acupuncture for chemotherapy-related nausea and vomiting. While somewhat less conclusive, the evidence also suggests that acupuncture may be useful against hot flushes, xerostomia, and pain. There are also promising results from pilot studies of acupuncture for cancer-related fatigue and chemotherapy-induced neutropenia and neuropathy, amongst other symptoms that acupuncture might be able to alleviate.[3]

References

1. Barrie R. Cassileth, MS, PhD, and Ian Yarett. Integrative Medicine Service, Memorial Sloan Kettering Cancer Center, New York.
2. Deng G, Seto D, Cassileth B. (2012) Recent clinical trials of acupuncture for cancer patients, in Cho WCS (ed): *Acupuncture and Moxibustion as an Evidence-based Therapy for Cancer: Evidence-Based Anticancer Complementary and Alternative Medicine*. Dordrecht, The Netherlands, Springer Science+Business Media.
3. Stone JA, Johnstone PA. (2010) Mechanisms of action for acupuncture in the oncology setting. *Curr Treat Options Oncol* **11**:118–127.

Rehabilitation Programs

Doctors and scientists have discussed and debated for many years about how the health and immunity of cancer patients can be preserved or improved. The effectiveness of rehabilitation program for cancer patients was discussed in an issue of the *Canadian Medical Association Journal* in 2014.[1] The key message was that the rehabilitation program resulted in better quality of life during chemotherapy for cancer patients. The key terms highlighted in this program were (1) exercise, (2) nutrition, and (3) symptom control (i.e., controlling the symptoms of side effects). The program aimed at mitigating the side effects of chemotherapy through symptom management, nutritional supplements, and health maintenance with exercise.

Reference

1. *Canadian Medical Association Journal*, July 24, 2014.

Pre-rehabilitation Programs — Rehabilitation Programs Prior to Surgery and Chemotherapy

Most patients go with a rehabilitation program after surgery to speed up the recovery process. One report[1] stated that patients who go for rehabilitation programs prior to surgery can recover even faster.

Pre-rehabilitation programs can especially benefit weaker or elderly patients. There was a clinical trial with 77 colorectal cancer patients who required surgery. They undertook a rehabilitation program which involved physical fitness training, aerobics, nutrition counselling with nutritionists, and consultations with psychologists to help with concerns and stress related to cancer treatment.

Half of the trial patients were assigned to the rehabilitation program approximately 25 days prior to surgery, while the other half started the rehabilitation program after surgery. A comparison of the two groups were made by testing the distance the patients could walk within 6 minutes, two months post-surgery.

Not surprisingly, the group assigned to prehabilitation did better on a presurgery test that measured how far they could walk in 6 minutes. Two months after surgery, the prehabilitation group walked an average of 23.7 meters farther than when they started the study. Rehab-only patients walked an average of 21.8 meters less than when they started. (A change of 20 meters is considered clinically significant.)

Reference

1. Dr. Julie Silver. A physiatrist at Spaulding Rehabilitation Hospital in Boston, *Journal Anesthesiology*. October 29, 2014.

Physical Therapists for Cancer Patients

Though many hospitals across the world have yet to utilize dedicated physical therapists for cancer patients, physical therapist services for cancer patients are already available in hospitals and cancer centres in the US. The presence of dedicated physical therapists is a great benefit to cancer patients and they help with improving patients' quality of life and prolonging their survival.

Once a patient is newly diagnosed with cancer, the patient will meet several people including doctors, nurses, physician assistants, and social workers.

During the course of anti-cancer medical treatments, cancer patients will face difficulties mainly due to adverse events (e.g., toxicities) from chemotherapy. Physical therapists belonging to the hospital's cancer care team provide unique and important services to cancer patients. For instance, they assess the physical condition of cancer patients and support them in solving any difficulties encountered. Let's learn more about the work of physical therapists.

Question 1: What is the role of a physical therapist in the treatment of cancer?[1]

People may think of a physical therapist as someone who takes care of sports-related injuries, like injury caused by impact to the muscle or bone. But a physical therapist in a cancer care team helps to rectify various functional problems in patients. The physical therapist can provide customized therapy to resolve physical difficulties in a patient's daily life, such as functional degradation in the heart, lungs, nerves, skin, pelvis, and inner ear.

Side effects from cancer treatment can be minimized by getting the patient to take part in physical strengthening programs before starting chemotherapy. During chemotherapy, the physical therapist can also help the patient maintain body strength and balance while reducing pain and fatigue by working on the patient's whole-body movements. On top of that, such physical therapy can also help patients smoothly go through the end of life period.

The physical therapist helps to bridge the gap between the doctor's orders and the patient's everyday life. With support from the physical therapist, patients will be able to understand the whole treatment process better, do better in self-management, and complete the cancer treatment safely and effectively.

Question 2: What is the most important thing that physical therapists can do for patients?[1]

The physical therapist should be able to identify their patients' needs by clearly understanding their condition and situation. They should listen to what the patients are saying and figure out what is important for them. They should help and encourage depressed cancer patients so that they can carry out their cancer treatment with confidence and a positive mind set.

Specific examples include helping a patient breathe better, helping a patient hug a family member, walking a patient on the street, or even jogging with a patient, all of which can help improve the patient's quality of life. The physical therapist can also help patients set small but concrete goals and help them achieve those goals. By doing so, the patient would feel that he or she is not alone in fighting the battle.

Question 3: How should a patient communicate with the physical therapist in order to get good physical therapy?[1]

Physical therapists will encourage patients to have an open mind and communicate with them about their fears and difficulties with cancer. Patients are encouraged to ask their physical therapists questions and discuss their expectations of the treatment and the possible difficulties that may be faced. Patients should also feel free to talk about their physical condition and describe how they feel physically (e.g., whether there is any discomfort experienced). Patients can directly contact physical therapists without recommendation from doctors.

The physical therapist can then consult the treating physician to see if there is any further medical advice or assistance needed.

In the US, you can find a physical therapist online at the American Physical Therapy Association website. The website lists a number of physical therapists in each region.

Reference

1. Sharlynn Tuohy, PT, DPT, MBA, Director of Rehabilitation at Memorial Sloan Kettering Cancer Center (MSKCC), and Jean Kotkiewicz, PT, DPT, CLT, Supervisor, Inpatient PT at MSKCC; September 23, 2014.

Cancer Diagnosis — Stress to Mental Illness

Being diagnosed with cancer is a devastating matter and can cause extreme stress. It will certainly impact the daily life of those diagnosed, and one third of such individuals will suffer from some form of serious mental illness such as depression.

Is it a real cancer? Why should I have cancer? What should I do from now on? Some patients may exhibit abnormal psychological behaviors, including blaming or cursing external parties. Compared to ordinary people suffering from daily stress, the mental state of new cancer patients is potentially much more unstable.

The psychological condition of cancer patients can degrade drastically due to excessive anxiety or persistent depression, thus preventing them from carrying out normal daily activities or maintaining healthy relationships with others. New cancer patients may need a doctor's prescription to alleviate the mental anxiety and stress.

The prognosis for breast cancer is usually better than other kinds of cancers, such as stomach cancer or pancreatic cancer which tend to be fatal. It is interesting to note that despite the better prognosis, breast cancer patients tend to experience greater anxiety compared to other types of cancer patients. Studies have shown that women are more emotionally sensitive to cancer compared to men, and women tend to express their feelings about

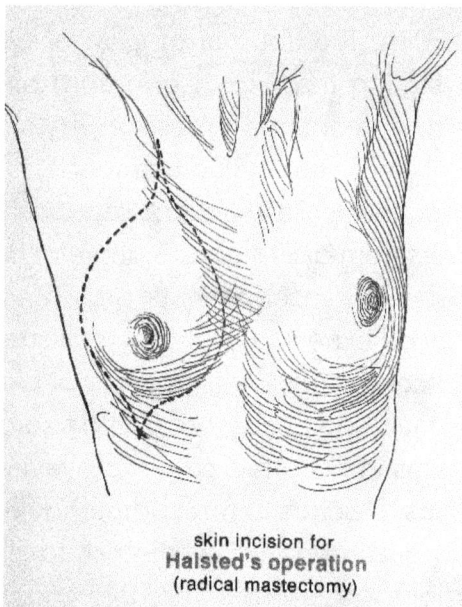

skin incision for
Halsted's operation
(radical mastectomy)

Picture of mastectomy.

cancer more openly. Mastectomy surgery for breast cancer patients can bring permanent changes to a woman's physical appearance, thereby causing even more concern or mental stress.

A paragraph cited from a novel shows deep frustration of a breast cancer patient: "My breast should be cut out. But I don't know how much breast should be removed or should the other side breast also be removed. Nobody, not even the doctor, seems to know about my breast and my cancer. Very lonely and gloomy journey to go through. How much time will I have, a few months or a year? Am I too greedy to think about a few more years?

Reference

1. Yeon Su Kim's novel, Girl at the end of the world.

Mitigating Mental Anxiety and Therapy for Cancer Patients

On 6 October 2014, the *Journal of Clinical Oncology* published a report stating that about one third of patients with cancer suffered from fear and depression. These patients also experienced problems with maladjustment.

It was reported that while 18 to 20% of ordinary people suffer some form of stress from daily life, 42% of breast cancer patients, 41% of head and neck cancer patients, and 39% of skin cancer patients experienced extremely high levels of stress. The report revealed that cancer patients suffer up to double the stress, in terms of both quantity and quality, compared to ordinary people.[1]

Medical teams in hospitals strive to alleviate these difficulties for patients. Doctors can recommend supportive programs such as group therapy, psychiatrist consultations, and counseling sessions that can provide help and guide patients on how to relieve stress.

It is said that 5 to 10 hours of counseling, psychological aid, or palliative care can be immensely useful for patients. These supportive programs can help patients understand that they are not alone, and that they can also overcome emotional stress by having a positive mindset.

But no matter how much the medical team tries to help, it will be up to the cancer patients who should try to overcome the difficulties related to the mental stress. A positive mindset would be a starting point for cancer patients to cope with emotional difficulties and mental suffering associated with cancer.

Reference

1. *Journal of Clinical Oncology*, Oct 6, 2014.

Points to Note Prior to Undergoing Breast Cancer Surgery

1. New guidelines for setting safe surgery margins for some breast cancers

The American Society of Clinical Oncology, Society of Surgical Oncology, and American Society for Radiation Oncology jointly issued a consensus guideline[1] on the margins for breast-conserving surgery with radiation for the treatment of women with ductal carcinoma in situ (DCIS).

DCIS is a breast cancer at a very early stage. This guideline was issued after a review of current practices involving about 7,900 patients. The use of a 2-millimeter margin as the standard for an adequate margin in DCIS, followed with whole breast radiation therapy, is associated with low rates of breast cancer recurrence. This new practice has the potential to decrease re-excision rates and improve cosmetic outcomes, resulting in an overall decrease in health care costs.

Reference

1. Society of Surgical Oncology, the American Society for Radiation Oncology, American Society of Clinical Oncology, News Release, Aug. 15, 2016.

2. The need for contralateral prophylactic mastectomy

Contralateral prophylactic mastectomy, or the removal of both breasts, is often performed even if there is a tumor in only one of the breasts. This is due to excessive concern and ultimately

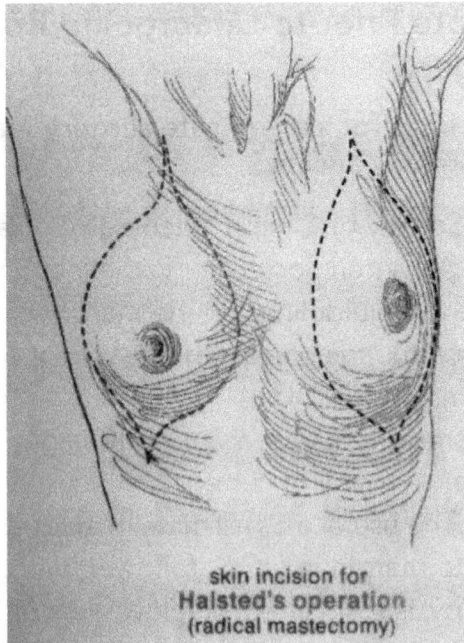

skin incision for
Halsted's operation
(radical mastectomy)

Contralateral prophylactic mastectomy — the removal of both breasts.

a misconception about breast cancer. Doctors who carry out contralateral prophylactic mastectomy believe that removing the other tumorless breast would help to prevent transition or metastasis of breast cancer.

However, as breast cancer patients learn more about the availability of different options for surgery, there is a gradual change away from opting for contralateral prophylactic mastectomies. It was reported that among breast cancer patients today, 59% had lumpectomy, 32% had unilateral mastectomy (the removal of only one breast), and only 9% had contralateral prophylactic mastectomy (the removal of both breasts).[1]

Reference

1. Katharine Yao, MD, Clinical Associate Professor of Surgery at Pritzker School of Medicine at University of Chicago, Abstract #71, Breast Cancer Symposium, September 4–6, 2014, San Francisco.

Chapter 8

Clinical Trials for Cancer Patients

The Drug Development Process and Clinical Trials

Plenty of work goes into the entire drug development process, which largely involves laboratory studies (basic research and laboratory tests), animal experiments (using several kinds of experimental animal models), and different phases of clinical trials (tests in humans). It is useful to understand the two key trials that underlie drug development.

- Pre-clinical trials — experiments carried out before testing in humans; this includes laboratory studies and animal testing.
- Clinical trials — drug under study given directly to humans after pre-clinical tests show that it is safe and potentially beneficial to proceed with human clinical trials.

Types of Clinical Trials

Clinical trials can be classified as follows:

- Bioavailability/Bioequivalent Trials — These trials are typically conducted for the development of generic drugs. Tests on humans are often carried out with the aim of determining the efficacy or safety of generic drugs in comparison to existing drugs in the market.

- Phase 1 Clinical Trials — The first-in-human clinical trials are carried out on a small number of healthy volunteers or patients using potential drug candidates that are qualified from pre-clinical trials. The main objectives of Phase 1 trials are to evaluate the safety (toxicity) of the drug and to determine the proper dosage of the drug to be used.

- Phase 2 Clinical Trials — These trials are aimed at evaluating the efficacy and safety of drugs with a bigger group of patients (approximately 50 to 200) based on data and insights obtained from Phase 1 trials.

- Phase 3 Clinical Trials — Phase 3 trials are conducted only after Phase 2 trials produce positive results. A global Phase 3 clinical trial with cancer drug usually requires the participation of 400–1,000 cancer patients. The number of patients needed for a clinical trial is dependent on the specific objectives of the clinical trial, the design of the study, and the statistical analysis to be conducted.

How are Clinical Trials Carried Out?

Pharmaceutical companies carry out clinical trials to evaluate the efficacy of their new drugs and to investigate the toxicity (i.e., side effects and adverse effects) of the drug on participating patients (i.e., the subjects). Clinical trials are designed based on protocols prepared by pharmaceutical companies and executed by research doctors at contracted hospitals. Experts from pharmaceutical companies and hospitals will do their best to protect the safety of subjects throughout the clinical trials.

All subjects in the clinical trial will be treated with study drugs according to the study protocol. And data (safety and efficacy) of subjects' response to the drugs during the clinical trial period will be collected. When the clinical trial is completed, the data collected will be statistically analyzed. The statistical analysis will determine if the new drug is superior to the comparator drug used in the study. Thus, the safety and efficacy of the new drug will be evaluated against the comparator drugs.

In accordance with the clinical trial protocol, clinical trials are subjected to regular monitoring and audits to ensure the safety of patients and the quality of data collected. The efficacy and safety data will also periodically be put through an objective evaluation by an independent third-party review committee.

As the clinical trial progresses, research staff must perform their responsibilities faithfully, carrying out all duties according to the clinical trial protocol, and collecting all records in a transparent manner.

Phase 3 clinical trials, sponsored by companies or organizations, are carried out with several parties. These parties include hospitals, clinical research organizations (CROs), clinical trial program and software system management companies, CT/MRI image analysis companies, patient bio-sample screening and analysis companies, drug procurement and supply companies, drug and bio-sample delivery companies, ethics committees, clinical trial data management and statistical analysis companies, and test equipment management companies.

As the conduct of clinical trials requires the contributions of a variety of professionals equipped with advanced scientific and medical knowledge, laboratory skills, legal and regulatory compliance knowledge and many other forms of expertise, the business of clinical trials forms a big industry.

Key Players Involved in the Conducting of Clinical Trials

- **Sponsor** — A sponsor is a pharmaceutical company that supports the conduct of clinical trials with protocol development and financial support. Final study reports are produced upon completion of clinical trials, and if the trials are successful, the sponsoring pharmaceutical company will try to obtain approvals from governments around the world to sell the new drug in the market.

- **Contract Research Organization (CRO)** — The CRO is a company with staff who are trained to work in accordance with the protocol. CRO staff are regularly dispatched to work alongside clinical trial researchers (e.g., hospital doctors/nurses) to monitor the use of anti-cancer drugs, observe patients' response to medication, conduct regular checkups and tests for patients, and check the accuracy of patients' medical records, etc. The CRO staff provides technical support to ensure that the patients' data is properly collected and the patients' safety is protected.

- **Data Management and Statistical Analysis** — Although independent companies specializing in data management and statistical analysis exist, most big CROs are capable of carrying out their own management of data and statistical analyses. Clinical trial patients' data are entered into computer databases from which comprehensive reports can be generated. These reports are then analyzed to check for statistical significance.

- **Site Management Organization** — The SMO manages a team of trained research coordinators who are dispatched to hospitals to provide support for doctors conducting clinical trials. They will follow the doctor's instructions to assist in administrative tasks related to the clinical trials and play a role in the documentation.

- **Hospitals, Clinical Research Physicians, and Research Nurses** — These professionals carry out clinical trials according to the protocol outlined by the sponsor. Information on the medication used, how the patients were managed, and patients' clinical data are then entered into the CRO's computer system. Clinical samples obtained from patients are analyzed in an external central laboratory or in a laboratory within the hospital.

- **Central Laboratory** — Central lab is the organization that tests or conducts analyses of bio-samples (blood, urine, tissues, etc.) from subjects participating in clinical trials.

- **Ethics Committee** — The ethics committee is responsible for reviewing all clinical trial materials and making a decision whether a particular trial should be approved or not. The ethics committee is made up of the hospital's clinical specialists and non-clinicians (e.g., lawyers, pastor, etc). The ethics committee may regularly review and check the status of ongoing clinical trials. If there are critical problems found in the clinical trials, the ethics committee has the authority to terminate the trial.

- **Logistics and System Management** — Logistics and system management companies provide a wide range of support services for all parties involved in the conduct of clinical trials, using computer software programs that can accurately capture clinical trial data.

- **CT/MRI Scan Analysis Services** — These companies partic-ipate in clinical trials by reviewing and analyzing the CT/MRI scans of patients obtained from the hospital. The company analyzes the tumor scans according to international standards of tumor growth and makes a judgment whether tumors are present or absent, or whether the cancer has spread. As such the third-party tumor scan analysis company can improve the accuracy of tumor imaging data analysis in clinical trials.

- **Clinical Drug Supply Management and Delivery** — These companies provide a service of study drug sourcing and delivery to the hospitals. Clinical trial drugs are delivered from manufacturing factories, wholesalers, or warehouses to hospital pharmacies based on specific time schedules under appropriate drug storage and delivery conditions. It is essential that the drugs are delivered on time so that patients can receive their medication during their visit to the hospital.

- **Clinical Patient Sample Collection and Delivery** — These companies work to ensure that the collection and delivery of patients' biological samples are on schedule and under designated storage conditions during transportation to specified laboratories for analysis.

Global Clinical Trials Standard — Good Clinical Practice

All institutions and companies involved in clinical trials should work and comply with the global clinical trial standards set by the International Harmonization Conference, which are referred to as Good Clinical Practice (GCP). The sponsor will have to bear the ultimate responsibility in ensuring that all parties comply with GCP standards. If any party has made critical errors or experiences some problem during the operation of the clinical trials, the sponsor will be responsible for resolving those issues.

Many of these complex services should be executed according to GCP regulations so as to ensure that good quality data is collected. Data quality must be checked and maintained on a regular basis while the clinical trial is being conducted.

Finally, when government authorities review the submitted data package, seeking for market approval, they will carry out inspections on the selected parties involved in the clinical trials before approving the drug. If there are any significant data quality concerns found during the review or inspection by government authorities, the market approval of new drug will be denied.

How are Patients Protected and Cared for during a Clinical Trial?

Clinical trials should be conducted in compliance with the various laws and regulations in place, namely (1) GCP, (2) each country's laws and regulations for clinical trials stipulated by government authorities, and (3) requirements and standards for conducting clinical trials established by each hospital's ethics committee. The primary objective of these laws and regulations is to protect patients from the beginning to the end of the clinical trials.

The laws and regulations for the development of new drugs are much more conservative and strict compared to those of other industrial or commercial acts. According to these laws and regulations, pharmaceutical companies must perform routine checks and audits to ensure the quality and integrity of the data collected from clinical trials.

As part of due diligence oversight by the government, government officials will review or inspect the clinical trial data and results in the submission package. If the data is found to have serious problems or violated any laws or regulations, then the new drug cannot be approved for sale in the market. Therefore, the conduct of clinical trials must closely abide by GCP guidelines, follow well prepared protocols, and ensure the safety of participants.

This kind of strictly regulated clinical trials can provide cancer patients an opportunity to get treated with innovative new drugs. As drugs under development are not available in the market yet, patients would not have a chance to get treated with the new drugs unless they participate in a clinical trial.

During a clinical trial, physicians and nurses will administer patients with the new medication in accordance with clinical study protocols. These protocols contain detailed descriptions on how to proceed with the trial and how to properly manage patients during the trial. As patients participating in clinical trials are treated precisely according to the protocol by physicians and nurses, they may actually receive better care and attention compared to ordinary patients treated in hospitals.

The side effects that arise from taking anti-cancer drugs in clinical trials are carefully managed during the entire period of the trial. When a patient participates in a clinical trial, the costs associated with the drug treatment and management of side effects are borne by the pharmaceutical company. Patients do not have to pay any medical fees to take a part in a clinical trial. This means that when a participating patient visits the doctor during the clinical trial period, the patient does not need to pay anything as all the fees for consultations and tests have been pre-paid by the sponsor company. In the unlikely event that patients experience side effects from clinical trial drugs leading to serious health damage or death, the sponsor will assist in filing insurance claims to compensate these patients or their families.

Not all Subjects will Get Treated with New Drugs in Clinical Trials

The purpose of clinical trials is to confirm the superiority of new drugs versus existing ones in the market. Hence, in a clinical trial, 50% of the patients will be treated with a currently available drug on the market (the control group) while the other 50% will be administered the new drug in development. This means that the probability of a patient getting treated with the new drug is 50%.

Most patients take part in double-blinded clinical trials where an unbiased computer system randomly assigns them to either the new drug or the comparator drug. Even after the trial is completed, both the doctor and the patient will not know which drug had been assigned to which patient. Only in special circumstances such as in cases of emergency where the identity of the drug is crucial for the next step of treatment will exceptions be made.

If a patient is no longer keen to participate in a clinical trial due to the 50% probability of getting treated with a currently marketed drug rather than the new drug, the patient has the freedom to drop out. However, as the new drug is still under clinical development and thus not available in the market yet, the patient will only be able to receive drugs that are currently sold in the market. Even if a participating patient gets treated with the comparator (i.e., currently marketed) drug, the hospital will still continue to provide good care and treatment for the patient according to protocols, and this typically includes free regular health checkups, blood tests, and CT/MRI scans to check for cancer recurrence during participation in the clinical trial.

In addition, clinical research physicians and nurses are tasked to manage clinical trial patients strictly based on clinical trial protocols. Hence, compared to general patients in hospitals, clinical trial patients can get more precise medical care as stipulated by the clinical trial protocols.

Regular Patient Checkups in Hospitals during Clinical Trial Periods

Clinical trial protocols require that patients meet with their investigating doctors at the hospital on a regular basis (at least once every two or three months) to check the status of disease.

Although these checkups are important for monitoring the status of patients' health and disease conditions, they are commonly perceived to be uncomfortable and time consuming. Patients who are concerned that these regular follow-up visits to the doctor during the clinical trial period will be too troublesome may consider not taking part in clinical trials.

Can Everybody Participate in a Clinical Trial?

Not everybody can participate in clinical trials. Once a patient has read the consent form and understood the terms and conditions for participating in the clinical trial, he or she must sign on the consent form. After signing the consent form, the hospital will carry out a patient eligibility screening test to determine if the patient is qualified to participate.

Various tests such as blood tests (e.g., blood chemistry, hematology), CT/MRI scans, tumor assessments, specific DNA genetic tests, tests of vital signs, and physical examinations will be carried out to determine whether the patient is eligible to take part in the clinical trial. Only when all the requirements stated in the inclusion and exclusion criteria (i.e., pass/fail standards) of the protocol are met, a qualified patients can participate in a clinical trial.

Before Consenting for Clinical Trial Participation

Based on what has been described so far, participation in a clinical trial appears more beneficial than we thought. Most of the time, cancer patients will follow the directions or recommendations of their doctors as to whether they should take part in clinical trials despite difficulties to understand the design and protocol of a clinical trial.

Cancer patients often face difficulties in consenting for clinical trials as doctors or nurses have limited time to explain the details of the clinical trials to them. It is not rare for a cancer patient to give consent to participate without fully understanding the details of the clinical trial. To understand the details of a clinical trial, it is imperative that patients should get help from experts who have scientific knowledge and experience in clinical trials. Other knowledgeable individuals, such as educated friends or family members of the patient, can also assist in to explaining the details of the clinical trial so that they can make an informed decision on whether to participate.

Types of Clinical Trials Available

There are many different types of clinical trials available from hospitals. Let's try to understand the various types of clinical trials that patients can join.

- **Early-stage clinical development (Phases 1 and 2) and late-stage clinical development (Phase 3)**

There are three phases of clinical trials conducted. Most of the time, drug development starts with Phases 1 and 2 clinical trials which involve a small number of patients. Phase 3 clinical trials, the last phase of development, are usually very large and may involve hundreds or thousands of patients.

In some cases, hospital doctors who are interested in doing some personal or independent research may approach some pharmaceutical companies for support. Such trials are usually small in scale and are known as investigator-initiated trials.

In terms of risk to patients, the toxicity profiles (i.e., adverse events) of drugs under study would be discovered during Phases 1 and 2. The safety of the studied drugs are usually well evaluated in the early phases before they can be moved on to Phase 3. Hence, Phase 3 studies would be less risky in terms of adverse events for patients compared to studies in the earlier stages.

If the cancer in a patient is still progressing or recurring despite treatment with currently available anti-cancer drugs, then the next best option for terminal-stage cancer patients would be to join an early-phase clinical trial and try a novel drug that has not been well tested yet but may give them a chance to improve their condition. In such circumstances, early-phase clinical trials, despite the uncertain risk of adverse effects, could still be beneficial for patients.

- **Extension of clinical indications of currently marketed drugs**

Once a new cancer drug has been approved for some particular indication (e.g., stomach cancer), the next step would be to check the effectiveness of this cancer drug for other indications (e.g., liver cancer, lung cancer, etc). For instance, to check if the indication of a stomach cancer drug may be extended to the treatment of liver cancer, the company should conduct another clinical trial using the drug which has already been approved for stomach cancer on liver cancer patients. As the stomach cancer drug has already been approved by government authorities, the risks of participation in the liver cancer trial would be low as the safety and efficacy profiles of the drug have already been established with the stomach cancer study.

- **New drugs that are already approved for sale in other developed countries**

Sometimes, there are new anti-cancer drugs that have been approved for sale in some countries but not yet in others. Hence, in order to obtain a country's approval to sell these anti-cancer drugs in their market, domestic clinical trials need to be conducted. The risk of taking part in these clinical trials should be low as the safety and efficacy of these drugs have already been established and the drugs have already been sold in other countries.

- **Global Phase 3 clinical trials**

Global pharmaceutical companies usually conduct multi-national Phase 3 clinical trials which simultaneously involve many hospitals in several countries. The data obtained from these global Phase 3 clinical trials will enable the registration of these new drugs in many countries at the same time. Before approving these clinical trials, each country's governing health authority and hospital ethics committees will carefully review the clinical trial protocols and check the risks and benefits for patients. Thus, the risk of joining a global Phase 3 clinical trial is usually on the low side.

- **Bio-equivalence tests**

Pharmaceutical companies that want to develop a generic drug product (i.e., a drug copy of an original one) should carry out bio-equivalence tests and get approvals from governing agencies such as the US Food and Drug Administration. Even though the degree of innovation may be lower, the efficacy and safety of these generic drugs will be equivalent to existing ones. Hence, participation in these trials should carry low risk.

- **Clinical trials using biosimilar drugs**

Biosimilar drugs are replications of existing antibody molecule drugs whose efficacies have been confirmed. These types of drugs are being developed by several biotechnology companies. As large molecule antibody drugs are very expensive and, in some cases, the cost may not be covered by the insurance, participation in clinical trials with biosimilar drugs should be beneficial to participating patients.

- **Clinical trials with placebo**

A placebo (non-drug) is sometimes used as a comparator to the new drug in development. This rare type of clinical trial is conducted if no standard drugs exist for a particular disease. In other words, there is no target drug that can be compared to in order to evaluate the new drug.

Patients who participate in placebo-controlled clinical trials will not know if they received the treatment drug or placebo. Most of these trials are double-blinded for both the patient and the doctor, and the assignment of either the drug or the placebo to participants is carried out by computer-assisted programs so as to reduce bias.

Although the patient will not know if he or she had taken the active drug or a placebo (at least for the duration of the clinical trial), participation can still be beneficial as there will be free-of-charge periodic medical checkups to monitor the health status of the patient. As soon as any signs of cancer recurrence or progression are detected during these regular medical checkups, the patient can swiftly acquire alternative drugs to treat the cancer. Nonetheless, placebo-controlled anti-cancer drug clinical trials usually have a lower rate of participation.

A Key Message

This chapter discussed the various types of clinical trials that are conducted and their associated risks and benefits. However, it is usually difficult to determine which types of clinical trials will be more beneficial or less risky to a patient. In every clinical trial, the drug profile and characteristics are different, and thus the benefits and risks of the drug to patients also vary. In addition, the cancer type and stage can vary from person to person. Hence, several critical points must be considered before patients decide to join a clinical trial.

Specifically, it is recommended that patients consider (1) the type and stage of their cancer, (2) the characteristics of the drug being tested, and (3) the type of clinical trials available.

In summary, patients who are financially capable will be able to buy medication that is available on the market, but unless they take part in clinical trials, they will not have the opportunity to get treated with innovative drugs that are under development. If you do participate in a clinical trial, you will have a chance of getting treated with an innovative new drug (the treatment group) or a currently marketed drug (the control group) without incurring any medical costs. However, the opportunity to take part in a clinical trial is limited by the qualification criteria that is defined in its protocol.

9 Quality of Life

Well-Being and Well-Dying

We have many difficult decisions to make throughout our lives. One of the most difficult things we will ever have to think about is how we prepare for death.

It is common that people prepare their wills in advance with endearing messages for their beloved ones and guidance on how their assets should be distributed upon death. Preparing for death, however, is not a simple process, like a flow chart with a straightforward "yes" or "no" decision algorithm. Apart from committing suicide, the process leading up to death can be quite complex and difficult to anticipate. Even with good planning, it will not be easy to face death when the time comes.

For most ordinary people, dealing with impending death is an unfamiliar matter. It is difficult to prepare in advance for death in some a systematic manner since people can die in various ways for various reasons.

Nevertheless, contemplation of death is important, and it is worthwhile to meditate on the inevitable pathway toward the end when we are physically and psychologically healthy.

Contemplation of Death

Though we don't recognize it, death exists closely at every moment of our daily life. However, it seems difficult to prepare for death in advance due to several aspects of our busy lives.

First, we have only been educated or trained to survive and sustain a good life in this world. In contrast, there is no guidance or training program available yet for people to prepare for dying well as they approach the end of life.

Second, we are always rushing towards building a better life, working diligently everyday, and surrounded by many busy people who are also pursuing their own activities. Thus, we are too much preoccupied with life's endeavors to think about death.

Third, people naturally prefer to avoid thinking about death. As living beings, people may be psychologically biased to believe that their life would go on forever. There is a song with the following lyrics: "though most people cannot live beyond a hundred years, they are acting like they can live for a thousand years; they don't see their death existing in the short life, but think that the death is somewhere far away on the other side of the Amazon River."

Nonetheless, dying is the final process that everyone must inevitably face some day in the future. Just as we invest our time and effort for better living, we should invest some time for studying and thinking in advance about death. The investment for studying the death will be enable us to go for an elegant exit at the end.

Perhaps the most optimal exit for a terminal patient would be being able to share the final farewell with loved ones in good consciousness.

It would be highly desirable for a patient to have some time to look back on his or her life, reconcile with others, and share affections with loved ones, rather than dying in unconsciousness on a hospital bed under excessive medical treatment.

When a patient is under excessive medical treatment during his or her final days, the patient's body is in the process of becoming more and more lifeless as the days go by, marked by increasing unconsciousness. Finally, when no more medical options can help sustain the patient's life, a body that never regains consciousness will mark the termination of life.

For the Sake of Some Final Consciousness

Is it worthwhile to maximize medical interventions for terminally ill patients to extend their life a little bit longer? Should the hospital not give up until all medical options have been exhausted, until the patient finally passes away? There will always be a struggle between the hope to live and the acceptance of death.

Perhaps it would be ideal if patients can decide for themselves how they would like to approach their impending end — whether to peacefully accept death or to struggle all the way to the end using all possible medical options available. However, it is difficult for cancer patients to make this decision without knowing if they are really reaching their final stages of life.

A patient would be able to make a better judgment if he or she can see the entire picture of his or her current health condition, understand the status of disease, and know the medical treatment options available. An objective assessment can be made based on an accurate assessment of the patient's cancer status and health condition with consultation from doctors and other experts.

As we have studied and worked hard to maintain a good life (well-being) since childhood, we should also learn how to prepare for an elegant death (well-dying). Just as studying hard for an examination in school brings good results, if we study, learn, and prepare for well-dying, then an elegant journey towards the end will be very possible for all of us.

So what should I do if I am judged to be taking my final steps in life? Should I do whatever it takes to try and prolong my survival, such as by taking other medical treatment options, embarking on yet another chemotherapy regimen, or by inserting tubes into mybody for feeding or breathing? Or should I just be calm and cool, and take a stroll towards the exit door at the end? Although the latter option might leave me with a little less time to live, it would help relieve me from the severe stress and costs that will arise from excessive medical treatment, and also help provide me with a better state of consciousness to spend my remaining time with family members and loved ones.

It is especially difficult for family members to make this decision of whether to continue fighting on or pulling the plug off on behalf of their loved one. It would therefore be better if the patients themselves can make the decision in advance on how they would like to be treated, thereby relieving the painful burden on both the patients themselves and their family members in their final days.

A Sober Evaluation for Wise Judgment

For chemotherapy at the onset of cancer as well as subsequent treatment after cancer recurrence, patients should do some risk and benefit assessments on the medical options available for disease treatment. Similarly, patients should also do a sober evaluation of the risk, costs, and benefits of medical treatments for the last days of their lives, focusing on the quality of life rather than meaningless extension of time just for breathing.

Risk — Consider a terminal-stage cancer patient going through excessive medical treatment, including taking on more cycles of chemotherapy. The patient's immune system might have already lost the strength to fight against the cancer cells. With additional chemotherapy, which is essentially a toxic cocktail of multiple drugs, the already weakened body will need to fight and tolerate the toxicities of chemotherapy in hopes of surviving just a little bit longer.

Cost — In addition to a deteriorated quality of life, the expenses incurred from excessive medical treatment will be a huge financial burden to the patient and his or her family. The cost of healthcare during the last periods of a patient's life can be 40 to 50% of what he or she will have spent in a lifetime. A careful weighing of the cost of excessive medical treatment to extend one's life against the quality of life is therefore an important matter.

Benefit — It is possible for last-stage cancer patients to live up to a few more weeks or months depending on their health condition and the availability of medical treatment options. While the possibility is very low, if they are very lucky to get treated with an appropriate novel drug that works perfectly for the disease, their life may be prolonged much longer.

Medical Treatment in the Final Stages and Human Dignity

An analysis of the medical cost incurred over a lifetime for the average person showed that medical costs during the last year of life accounts for approximately 40 to 50% of the entire cost. The highest profit returns for hospitals, pharmaceutical groups, and medical device companies come from the "business" of dying, which includes the intensive medical treatments during patients' last stage of life.

Let's take look at why such a large amount of medical spending occurs at the last stage of life. A key causing factor is based on the professional mission of hospitals and medical doctors to fight all diseases and save patients' lives with all medical means available.

Does this mission always justify the use of excessive medical treatment for last-stage cancer patients? Excessive medical treatment used to extend the life will include not-yet tried drugs, up-titrating the dose of anti-cancer medication, carrying out more surgeries, and using various high-tech equipment available.

It is, however, not just the hospitals or medical doctors who are solely responsible for these excessive medical treatments. The responsibility should also be on the patients themselves or their family members in deciding whether more medical treatments are needed.

How would a patient's final stage of life be like under intensive and excessive medical treatment? Their quality of life will drastically deteriorate due to the stressful side effects of excessive treatment. Family members who continue to take care of the terminal-stage patient will also be stressed in addition to the heavy financial burden they have to take on.

Perhaps the most important point to think about is the loss of dignity of the dying person. To desperately extend one's life without certainty of how long it will last, all possible medical interventions could be used, albeit resulting in intolerable stress to one's body. The patient will then gradually lose not only their consciousness but also their personal dignity as he or she is turning into a lifeless body mass, just for the sake of breathing for a little while longer. In this struggle to extend life, the patient will fade out little by little of their intelligence, emotion, memories, and soul. In this state of deterioration, the personal ability to react to any stimulation will be lost and only a body with no consciousness will be left, and then the body with no consciousness will be dying eventually after a few days or weeks.

Thus, it is recommended to carefully consider the quality of life and personal dignity during the course of dying. It will be better to make a decision, when you are in healthy condition, of which way to choose, either excessive treatment to extend life for a while, or accepting the end with conscious time to say good bye. It's a critical matter whether you will make a decision of the way of your own death or your death to be decided by somebody else.

Chapter 10 Hospice and Palliative Care

In 1974, New Haven Hospital in Yale was the first hospital to implement a hospice facility for terminally ill patients in the US. Since then, many countries around the world have also started hospice facilities and programs.

A hospice provides terminal-stage patients with comfortable end-of-life care, which includes pain relief treatment and counseling instead of excessive medical treatments to extend life.

Some Suggestions for the Improvement of Hospices

According to an article published in the *Journal of Palliative Medicine* on 7 August 2014, there were some difficulties and issues with hospice service providers in the US.

One third of the patients using hospice facilities in the US have stopped receiving their services or left from the hospice facilities. The 33 % eviction rate from hospice facilities implied that there were either some serious problems with hospice programs or ethical issues with the founders of hospice facilities.

In the US, the eviction rate of hospice facilities operated by private companies is two times higher than that of public facilities. The reasons for premature evictions are (i) inappropriate facilities, (ii) issues related to the quality of care, and (iii) the enrolment of patients who are not terminally ill.

According to the rules set by US Medicare, a hospice facility should only accept patients with a life expectancy of less than 6 months, and the mission of the hospice is not to carry out medical treatments for patients but to help patients relieve physical and mental pain in their final days.

However, there are often unexpected costs incurred from unnecessary tests and prescriptions for the patients. Some hospices even send patients to the hospital emergency room to die in an attempt to reduce their costs and workload.

The US Federal Government is constantly investigating fraudulent insurance claims from hospices. The total amount of suspicious insurance claims from US hospice facilities may reach US$1 billion.

Aside from the issue of cost, another problem is that some hospice facilities may accept patients who can live longer than 6 months and administer them with strong pain relief drugs or other forms of narcotics. A toxic cocktail of medications can often shorten the lives of these patients.

Over the past 10 years, the number of private hospice facilities has increased significantly in the US. In 2000, about 30% of hospices were operated by private companies while the other 70% were operated by local government organizations, religious groups, or non-profit organizations. However, in 2012, the proportion of hospices operated by private enterprises rose to 60%. As the number of privately operated hospices increased, so did the number of insurance claims and the eviction rate of patients.

The business of dying appears to reap good profits for private companies, but it may also lead to many complex social issues. It is important to learn more details about hospice services before selecting a hospice facility to register with.

When is a Right Time to Get Hospice Service[1]?

In 2013, 1.5 million patients in the US received care from hospices, of whom one third passed away within a week of commencing hospice care. This means that many patients start receiving hospice care only when it is too late.

Research shows that, among patients who received hospice care, 34.5% received less than 7 days of care and 50% received less than 18 days of care. Among the total number of patients in the US, 66% received care at nursing homes or their own homes rather than hospices. Medicare insurance covered 91% of the costs associated with hospice care services.

Another issue is the misconception that hospice care is only for cancer patients. In fact, 63% of hospice patients suffer from diseases other than cancer, such as dementia, heart disease, respiratory disease, and renal disease, just to name a few.

Reference

1. US National Hospice and Palliative Care Organization; J. Donald Schumacher, President and CEO of the National Hospice and Palliative Care Organization, November 3, 2014.

Hospice Services at the Hospital

A survey was conducted on staff working at cancer centers in the US, asking if it is possible for terminal-stage patients to die with dignity in hospitals. Fifty percent of the staff working at cancer centers answered "yes, it is possible" while 95% of the staff working at palliative care centers said that patients can die with dignity in hospital wards.

Although most patients would prefer dying at home, most of them pass away at either nursing homes or hospitals. If it is difficult for patients to make a trip home or if they do not like to be transferred to a new and unfamiliar place like a nursing home with new people around, it would be better for them to remain at the same hospital and receive continuous care from familiar staff. To provide patients with comfortable hospice care services at hospitals, the hospitals should keep staff well trained with good quality hospice service programs.

Hospice Palliative Care at Home Using an Automated Symptom-Monitoring Telephone System

More than 80% of people are dying away from home. People may wish to stay and die at home peacefully, but they are passing away somewhere else without fulfilling their last wishes. It is neither easy nor practical for terminal-stage patients to receive hospice palliative care at home.

There was a report of a home hospice care program that was successfully carried out using a remote automated system to enable better observations and provide real-time coaching to family caregivers. In the study,[1] 243 family hospice caregivers for terminal stage cancer patients were monitored daily using an automated symptom-monitoring telephone system. By random assignment, 119 family caregivers tried the unique symptom care intervention and 124 family caregivers provided normal care. All family caregivers in the intervention group called in to the monitoring system daily, reporting on a scale of 0 (none) to 10 (a lot) the presence of 11 common patient symptoms in the past 24 hours as well as their own fatigue, hours of sleep, mood, and the level of anxiety.

The study team analyzed the data collected on the 11 different symptoms. The surveyed symptoms are pain, shortness of breath, diarrhea or constipation, urination, change in thinking, nausea or vomiting, fatigue, depression, anxiety, insomnia, and poor appetite. The most common symptoms observed were fatigue (70%), pain (64%), poor appetite (54%), anxiety (39%), and change in thinking (38%).

The analyzed data showed that patients' symptom severity levels were highly correlated with their family caregivers' level of distress. The data also indicated that the vitality of family caregivers was better in the group that used the automated symptom-monitoring telephone system compared to the normal care group. This study provided preliminary evidence that such remote automated systems can be beneficial for family caregivers providing end-of-life care to patients at home.

The purpose of a hospice is to provide terminal-stage patients with comfortable end-of-life care which includes pain-relief treatment and counseling. To effectively help terminal-stage patients and caregivers working in either homes, nursing homes, or hospitals, a well prepared and standardized guidelines would be needed.

Reference

1. Bob Wong, Ph.D. Director of Applied Statistics, College of Nursing, University of Utah, 2014 Palliative Care in Oncology Symposium; Abstract 85, presented Oct 24, 2014.

End-of-life Care Discussions may Miss Patient Priorities[1]

A survey was carried out on more than 200 elderly Canadian patients who have been hospitalized with serious illnesses and 205 of their family members, asking them about the importance of 11 recommended elements in end-of-life care. The top five end-of-life issues that are missing during discussions with doctors are:

1. Care preference in the event of life-threatening illness
2. Patient values
3. Prognosis of the illness
4. Fears and concerns
5. Opportunity to ask additional questions regarding care

Patients and their family members felt that they did not have enough time and discussions with doctors. Only an average of 1.4 out of the 11 recommended elements in end-of-life care get discussed during the first few days of admission into hospital. The author of the study reported that the more elements in end-of-life care that doctors discussed with patients, the more satisfied patients and their family members about the care experience. The findings can guide improvements to end-of-life communication and decision-making in hospital settings.

Reference

1. Dr. John You, Associate Professor of Medicine, and Clinical Epidemiology and Biostatistics at McMaster University in Hamilton, Ontario, CMAJ (Canadian Medical Association Journal), November 3, 2014.

Eight Different Symptoms Observed in Terminal-Stage Cancer Patients Facing an Impending Death[1]

Researchers monitored the physical changes of more than 350 advanced-stage cancer patients and identified eight physical signs in patients who were facing death within a few days. These signs can also be observed by doctors, nurses, and family caregivers at the bedside. Better awareness of these telltale signs can help family members and caregivers anticipate an impending death and make better choices for end-of-life care.

The eight symptoms observed are:

1. Inability to close eyelids
2. Diminishing ability to react to visual stimulation
3. Reduced ability to react to sounds and words
4. Facial drooping
5. Non-reactive pupils
6. Hyperextension of the neck (causing the head to tilt further back when lying down)
7. Vocal cord grunting
8. Bleeding in the upper digestive tract

The report says that most patients will exhibit these symptoms three days before death. Although there are exceptions sometimes, these symptoms are nonetheless generally instructive for doctors and caregivers who have to make decisions during end-of-life care.

References

1. David Hui, MD, Assistant Prof. Dept of Palliative Care and Rehabilitation Medicine, University of Texas MD Anderson Cancer Center, Huston; R. Sean Morrison, MD Director, Lilian and Benjamin Hertzberg Palliative Care Institute, Mount Sinai Icahn School of Medicine, NY city Cancer Online, February 9, 2015.
2. R. Sean Morrison, (2015) MD. Director, Lilian and Benjamin Hertzberg Palliative Care Institute, Mount Sinai Icahn School of Medicine, NY city, *Cancer* Online.

Chapter 11

Healthcare Policies for Patients

Service Quality Assessments of Hospitals and Physicians

Healthgrades.com was started in the US in October 2014. This program gives the end users of medical services (i.e., patients) the opportunity to evaluate physicians and hospitals on specific disease categories and shares these evaluations with the public. The evaluation items include:

- The level of experience of doctors
- The medical service quality of doctors
- The education and training records of doctors
- The working intensity of physicians (for example, 20% of doctors in hospitals may be responsible for 80% of the patients, resulting in short consultation time for patients)
- Unnecessary medical treatments or tests which may result in excessive medical costs

Healthgrades.com provides patients with good information to review and get better medical services. Furthermore, the program motivates doctors and hospitals to provide better service and upgrade themselves with the most recent medical information and technology.

The expansion and adoption of such information sharing systems is highly recommended for all states and countries as it ensures that doctors and hospitals maintain high standards in medical practice and services.

Palliative Care[1]

What is the palliative care? Whenever this question is asked, many people will reply that palliative care is the professional care given by physicians and nurses to patients who are dying. However, this is not the correct answer. Patients or family members usually do not fully understand what goes on in palliative care, and sometimes even doctors may not correctly understand palliative care.

If you request for palliative care from doctors, they will usually suggest that you do not need it since you are still good and will not die soon.

However, palliative care can be an important additional source of support in the treatment of serious disease and is not simply some way to mitigate pain for patients who are doomed to die.

By itself, palliative care increases the quality of medical services to patients as well as the family. It can also help to reduce the frequency of emergency hospitalizations for patients, thereby reducing related medical costs.

In the US, hundreds of thousands of doctors, nurses, and social work volunteers are trained with palliative care knowledge and skills.

Reference

1. Wall Street Journal, Health Care, Barbara Sadick, September 14, 2014.

Hospitals, Nursing Homes, and my Home

Most patients would like to live out their final days at home. They would want to be surrounded by family members and their favorite things, such as their books, music, pictures, and garden.

However, upon discharge from the hospital, terminal-stage cancer patients will be sent to nursing homes or hospices rather than home due to difficulties in getting appropriate care at home. Patients who are in less critical condition will also go through rehabilitation programs at the nursing home rather than be sent home. When their disease status worsens at the nursing home, they will go back to the hospital again and so forth to the nursing home or hospice. Thus, the chance that these patients can go back home for a long period of time is quite low.

To enable patients to stay home for their final months, weeks, or days, a standard home care system must be developed with with a guidance manual so that late-stage patients can be cared for at home, or wherever they wish to be. More professional home caregivers should be trained with a certified program prepared by the government or medical community.

Caregivers

One of the big difficulties faced by late-stage cancer patients is the use and cost of caregivers. Unless the patient has comprehensive medical insurance or national health insurance which pays for caregiver service fees, the cost can be a huge burden for most ordinary people. It is recommended that a standardized professional care program and system be developed and implemented to provide patients with affordable and well-trained caregivers. Another challenge is finding well-trained caregivers who can provide quality service.

Many countries with low-cost medical care systems do not have well-prepared programs or organizations to train and produce quality caregivers. To increase the availability of and provide well-trained caregivers for patients, a standardized professional care system should be implemented to train and manage caregivers.

12 Assessment of the Risk/Benefit/Cost of Medical Treatments

What Constitutes Excessive Medical Treatments and How Should They be Dealt with?

Excessive medical treatments for terminal-stage cancer patients will significantly increase healthcare costs while decreasing their quality of life. Despite the irony of this practice, it still frequently occurs in many hospitals or care centers to extend the life of terminal stage cancer patients.

Some key items that may constitute, underlie, or contribute to excessive medical treatments are:

- Misconception of "more is better" — patients' perception is that it is good to get more medical tests, examinations, and various therapeutic treatment of drugs;
- Overly protective medical services from physicians and hospitals;
- Financial incentives that follow with more medical treatments;
- Patient's desperate desire to get treated with every possible service available and to resolve all difficulties;
- Direct marketing to patients.

It is human nature to want to get cured with treatment using the best drug and medical tools available, leaving no room for regret. Similarly, doctors have strong motivations to fight and cure the disease for patients.

To avoid unnecessary excessive medical treatments, it is recommended for patients to do risk/benefit/cost assessment based on information and feedback available from experts and doctors to get the most beneficial treatment option.

An Example of Excessive Treatment for Prostate Cancer Patients

Most prostate cancer patients around 66-79 years old receive intensive medical treatments even though their remaining life expectancy is less than 10 years. If prostate cancer patients with less than a decade of life left receive intensive chemotherapy treatment, the risk would be higher than the benefit. In spite of this, aggressive radiation therapy following surgery is commonly carried out for prostate cancer patients.

However, intensive medical treatments are not recommended for prostate cancer patients. Results of clinical studies studies showed that there was no difference in overall survival periods between the patient group with aggressive medical treatment and the patient group with close watching and no treatment.[1]

Aggressive medical treatments may not extend the prostate cancer patients' survival period and yet decrease their quality of life due to toxicities from chemotherapy or radiation therapy. The common adverse effects caused by chemotherapy or radiation therapy for these prostate cancer patients include erectile dysfunction, difficulty of controlling urination, and difficulty with bowel movements. In addition to these adverse side effects, there will also be more financial burdens for the patient to bear.

Nonetheless, due to overestimations of survival time, excessive medical treatments for prostate cancer patients are currently still eagerly pursued. Furthermore, patients also want to get treated aggressively because they want to be relieved from the haunting distress that there might still be remnants of cancer in the body.

Doctors may have some data to predict the remaining life expectancy of patients based on their age. However, no accurate method yet exists to predict the remaining life expectancy of prostate cancer patients, though it would be dependent on their age and health conditions.

Therefore, before starting any anti-cancer therapy, it is recommended that doctors and patients do a precise evaluation of the risk and benefit of available treatments while considering the patients' age and health conditions. By doing so, cancer patients will be able to receive optimal medical treatments, avoiding excessive medical treatments.

Reference

1. Timothy J. Daskivich, MD, MSHPM, of the University of California Los Angeles, *Cancer*, 2014.

Five Important Points to Increase the Quality and Value of Cancer Treatment

As discussed, many doctors are willing to go beyond what is necessary to treat cancer patients and prolong their life by using all available medical armamentarium. This attitude will influence the desire of patients to get treated with new drugs or take up other forms of medical care, even if new treatments have not been proven to be effective and cause additional medical expense. Furthermore, more cycle of chemotherapy treatment will lead to deterioration of the patient's health.

The following are five common types of treatment and care that are unnecessary but commonly prescribed[1]:

1. Chemotherapy for terminal-stage cancer patients who will not be able to benefit from the chemotherapy (in this case, it would be better to use palliative care or symptom-relief care instead);
2. CT, PET, and bone CT scans for early-stage breast cancer patients to classify cancer types;
3. CT, PET, and bone CT scans for early-stage prostate cancer patients to classify cancer types;
4. Regular or frequent examinations of blood biomarkers with CT, PET, and bone CT scans for breast cancer patients who are under treatment and show no symptoms of cancer recurrence;
5. The use of G-CSF, a white blood cell-stimulating factor, for patients with low risk of febrile neutropenia (development of fever due to a deficiency in neutrophils).

Patients and doctors should try to avoid the unnecessary tests or treatments listed above as much as possible.

Reference

1. Dr. Lisa Hicks, MD, St. Michael's Hospital, University of Ontario, and Dr. Allen S. Lichter, CEO of ASCO, April 4, 2012.

Risk/Benefit/Cost Assessment

The cost of cancer care has risen enormously in recent years, with an average cost of at least $10,000 per month, or more than $30,000 per months in some cases. It would be good to do a risk/benefit/cost assessment before starting a certain cancer treatment. Even during treatment that is already underway, doing reassessments can help to increase the benefit versus the risk or cost.

To do a good risk and benefit assessment, patients need to have a clear understanding of their own cancer type and status as well as the medical options available for them. A stepwise assessment will be needed in this journey starting from the diagnosis of cancer, surgery, chemotherapy, rehabilitation and recovery, a healthy return to everyday life, the recurrence of cancer, cancer re-treatment, quality of life, hospice and palliative care, and finally death. A precise assessment is needed at each critical step.

While hospitals and physicians can be a great help, patients should also acquire knowledge about their cancer and the treatment plan so that they can go through the treatment process effectively and thus not only survive longer but also maintain a good quality of life.

Recently, the American Society of Clinical Oncology updated their value framework with a methodology to compare the clinical benefits, side effects, and costs of treatment regimens.[1] The value framework relies on high-quality data from randomized clinical trials including clinical outcomes and toxicity.

Data on the clinical benefits and side effects of each regimen are used to calculate an overall "net health benefit" (NHB) score. The NHB represents the added benefit that patients can expect from new therapy treatment versus current standards of care. The NHB is calculated based on data of improvements to overall or progression-free survival and the number and severity of toxicities. The NHB is presented along with the patient's expected out-of-pocket costs for the regimens being compared, as well as the overall drug acquisition cost.

Ultimately, what constitutes "value" will depend on what is personally important for each patient, such as length of life, quality of life, or affordable treatment.

Reference

1. ASCO Looking To Help Patients Assess Value of Cancer Therapy, by PPN Staff.

Chapter 13
Cancer Risk, Signs and Symptoms, Detection, and Support

Obesity, Post-Menopause, and Breast Cancer

White adipose tissue inflammation is defined by the presence of dead or dying adipocytes surrounded by an envelope of macrophages. The shape of this inflammation has been described as "crown-like structures of the breast" (CLS-B) and occurs mostly in obese women.

A study[1] showed that CLS-B occurrence and number of CLS-B/cm² are higher in overweight and obese patients versus lean patients, and in postmenopausal patients versus premenopausal patients. This means that white adipose tissue inflammation in the breast is associated with both increased body mass and menopause.

White adipose tissue inflammation in the breast is also related to an increase of aromatase activity, which is directly related to the occurrence of breast cancer and its growth. These findings therefore indicate that there will be an increased risk of breast cancer in overweight and post-menopausal women.

Reference

1. Neil M. Iyengar, M.D. The Memorial Sloan Kettering Cancer Center in New York City; American Society of Clinical Oncology's 2014 Breast Cancer Symposium, September 4–6, 2014.

Image courtesy of Blausen Medical

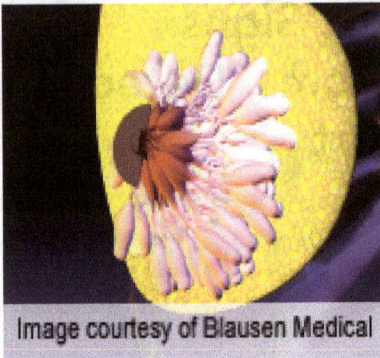

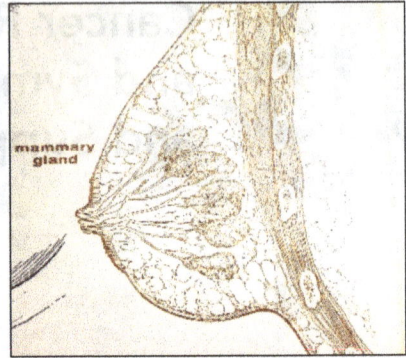

Image of crown-like structures of the breast (CSL-B).

Bra Wearing and Breast Cancer Risk[1]

Between 2007 to 2008, a team of researchers surveyed over 1,500 postmenopausal women aged 55 to 74 to see if there was any relationship between bra wearing and the occurrence of breast cancer.

Their results showed that there was no difference in breast cancer risk between women who regularly wore bras and women who did not wear bras, thus confirming that wearing bras will not cause breast cancer.

Reference

1. Cancer Epidemiology, Biomarkers & Prevention, September. 2014.

Ovarian Cancer Risk in Women Who Douche

It has been known that douching, or vaginal washing with a device, is associated with yeast infections, pelvic inflammatory disease, and ectopic pregnancies. According to the Office on Women's Health at the US Department of Health and Human Services, douching can cause an overgrowth of harmful bacteria, lead to yeast infection, and push bacteria upwards into the uterus, fallopian tubes, and ovaries. In addition, several reports have documented associations between douching and cervical cancer, reduced fertility, HIV, and other sexually transmitted diseases.

A new study report[1] from National Institute of Environmental Health Sciences study with more than 41,000 women reported that ovarian cancer risk is also associated with the douching procedure routinely practiced by millions of American women.

Reference

1. *Epidemiology*, online June 20, 2016.

Lack of Sleep and Prostate Cancer Risk

A study from the American Association for Cancer Research reported in 2017 that men younger than 65 who slept just three to five hours a night were 55% more likely to develop fatal prostate cancer than those who got seven hours of sleep a night, and six hours of sleep a night was linked to a 29% higher risk of prostate cancer death compared to seven hours. The study results are based on an analysis of long-term data on more than 823,000 men in the US led by Susan Gapstur, vice president of epidemiology at the American Cancer Society.

The authors stated that circadian rhythms, the body's natural sleep/wake cycle, might play a role in prostate cancer development. Lack of sleep can inhibit the production of melatonin, which is known to regulate sleep-wake timing and blood pressure and also plays a role as an antioxidant in the protection of nuclear and mitochondrial DNA. Melatonin also interacts with the immune system as low melatonin production can lead to an increase in genetic mutations, greater oxidative damage, reduced DNA repair, and a weakened immune system. Lack of sleep may also contribute to the disruption of genes involved in tumor suppression.

This finding serves to underscore the importance of having adequate hours of sleep to maintain good health.

Reference

1. American Association for Cancer Research, news release, April 3, 2017.

Vasectomy and Prostate Cancer Risk

Many men around the world have considered getting a vasectomy as birth control. However, concerns about the risk of prostate cancer with vasectomies has existed since the results of a Harvard Health Professionals study that was published in 1993. The study reported that men who had undergone vasectomies were about one and half times more likely to develop prostate cancer than men who did not do the procedure.

Since 1993, more studies have been conducted but failed to find a relationship between vasectomies and prostate cancer risk. The authors of these studies also could not establish a biologically plausible reason for why vasectomy might increase the risk of prostate cancer.

A study that was recently published in the *Journal of Clinical Oncology* in 2017 also showed that there was no elevated risk of prostate cancer among men who had undergone a vasectomy. This result is consistent with other studies, including the Cancer Prevention Study II which found no link between vasectomies and prostate cancer risk.

The American Urological Association currently agrees that vasectomy does not increase the risk of prostate cancer.

Reference

1. *Journal of Clinical Oncology*, March 2017.

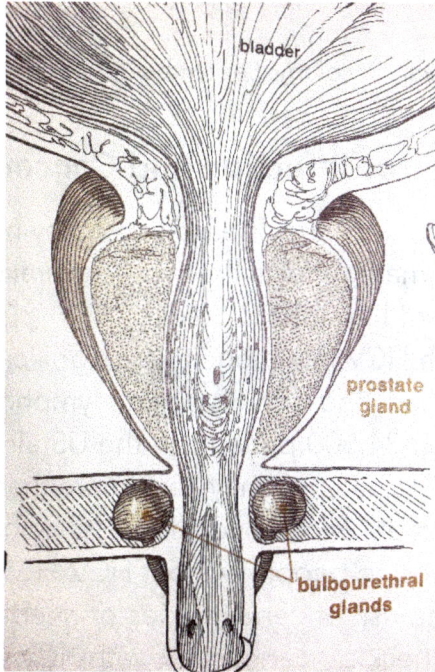

Anatomy of prostate gland. (*From Mellnoi's Illustrated Medical Dicition-ary*, The Williams & Wilkins Company.)

Baldness and Prostate Cancer Risk

Is there any relationship between baldness and prostate cancer? In 2014, the National Cancer Institute published an article in *Journal of Clinical Oncology* which recommended that men who had become bald by the their mid 40s should do a check for prostate cancer.

The report said that the risk of prostate cancer is 39% higher in men who had lost massive amounts of hair at the front or central parts of the scalp. The study also indicated that there was an elevated risk of prostate cancer in aging individuals who are also balding. It is recommended that elderly people with baldness should go for prostate cancer checks on a regular basis.

Reference

1. *Journal of Clinical Oncology*, September 2014.

Hepatitis C Virus Infection and Cancer Risk

Hepatitis C is an infectious disease caused by hepatitis C virus (HCV), which primarily affects the liver. Antiviral drugs can cure more than 90% of hepatitis C cases.

People with HCV infection have a significantly increased risk of liver cancers and non-Hodgkin's lymphoma. An analysis[1] of more than 34,500 patients in the US also showed that patients with HCV infection may have more than twice the risk of mouth and throat cancers and a five-fold higher risk of larynx cancers compared to people without HCV. HCV infection may also increase the risk of certain types of head and neck cancers. Head and neck cancer patients with HCV were also more likely to have HPV, which is related to several other types of cancer. HCV affects not only the liver but the rest of the body as well. HCV can also affect how cancer patients respond to anti-cancer treatment.

Blood transfusion, transfusion of blood products, or organ transplants without HCV screening can carry high risk of HCV infection. The screening of blood donors at a national level is therefore very important. The use of new needles and syringes can significantly decrease the risk of hepatitis C in intravenous drug users.

Reference

1. *Journal of the National Cancer Institute*, April 13, 2016.

Can the Signs or Symptoms of Cancer be Recognized?

Many middle-aged people may experience various common symptoms of cancer but they do not recognize them as serious symptoms of disease like cancer. Some symptoms that may imply the possible presence of cancer are coughing, bleeding, frequent changes in the status of faeces and urine, and weight loss. These symptoms were reported and listed in the journal *PLOS One* in December 2014.

The research team presented a survey[1] to 4,858 people aged above 50 who visited a hospital but did not have any cancer examinations done before. The questionnaire asked them questions about some uncomfortable symptoms experienced without mentioning or implying anything about cancer.

Out of the 4,858 people, 1,724 (35%) responded to the survey, and 915 out of the 1,724 respondents (53%) said they had experienced at least one or more of the listed symptoms in the past three months.

It would be premature to say that the people who experienced these symptoms must have cancer. Nonetheless, as these symptoms indicate a chance of disease, it would be worth going for a medical check when such symptoms are experienced to see if there is any cancer at the early stages.

Reference

1. Katriina Whitaker, Attributions of Cancer 'Alarm' Symptoms in a Community Sample, December 2, 2014, Doi: 10.1371/journal.pone.0114028.

Cancer Diagnosis Using Innovative Nano-Sensors

A variety of molecular biology techniques and methods, including biomarkers, are used for the diagnosis of cancer. Recently, the accuracy of diagnoses has improved significantly; however, there are still limits to detecting cancer with simple medical devices or armamentarium.

In September 2014, a report[1] introduced a very interesting cancer-detection method which is currently under development. The research team at Penn Vet Working Dog Center developed a kit for cancer diagnosis based on their findings with McBaine dogs. The research team prepared a set of 12 blood plasma sample tubes in which the 11th tube had a trace amount of cancer tissue mixed with plasma. It was found that the dogs could use their sense of smell to accurately detect the tube containing the trace amount of cancer tissue.

Using this insight, the institute is developing a "nano-sensor" to detect cancer. The technology is a very tiny sensor that can detect the smell of chemical ingredients emitted from cancer tissues, just like how the dogs smelled and detected the chemicals. Currently, chemists and physicists are collaborating with the study team to make nano-sensors that can detect trace amounts of cancer tissue that are as small as 1/100,000 the size of a hair diameter.

Reference

1. US Penn Vet Working Dog Center, September 2014.

Ovarian Cancer Detection by DNA Analysis of Vaginal Fluid

There were 22,000 women diagnosed with ovarian cancer in the US and it was estimated that 14,300 ovarian cancer patients would die in 2014. The mortality risk is higher in patients who were diagnosed with the cancer after menopause and patients who have a family history of ovarian cancer.

Ovarian cancer can be cured if it is detected and treated early. However, many ovarian cancers are diagnosed only after the cancer had already progressed significantly, and thus only 44% of ovarian cancer patients survived five years after the cancer was detected (Source: American Cancer Society). As ovarian cancer is not a common, there is no accurate diagnostic test available yet.

Although there are some symptoms for early-stage ovarian cancer, they do not serve as good indicators as they are not dis-ease-specific. For example, women might experience abdominal bloating or urinary problems, but these symptoms can also be caused by health problems other than ovarian cancer.

According to a recent research report,[1] it may be possible to detect ovarian cancer from gene mutations from vaginal fluid samples. Specifically, the researchers believe that ovarian cancer DNA can be detected from vaginal fluid as they were able to detect the tumor DNA in tampons used by several women with advanced ovarian cancer.

It would be very beneficial if a diagnostic kit can be developed to detect specific tumor DNA from vaginal fluid samples of early-stage ovarian cancer patients someday in the future, leading to more effective treatment.

References

1. Dr. David Mutch, professor of obstetrics and gynecology at Washington University in St. Louis.
2. Dr. Charles Landen, gynecologic cancer specialist at the University of Virginia in Charlottesville, November 2014 issue of *Obstetrics & Gynecology*.

Pre-cancer Cells Existing in Blood

About 140,000 people are diagnosed with blood cancers every year in the US. As explained in Chapter 1, the onset of cancer starts from gene mutations in cells. Most gene mutations are not inherited from parents but instead occur due to various external factors like stress, smoking, alcohol, and environmental toxins. As people age, they accumulate multiple mutations which may eventually lead to the onset of cancer when their immune system is weakened and unable to protect them.

Two independent studies[1] which carried out DNA analyses on approximately 30,000 people reported that pre-cancer cells commonly exist in our blood. While it is rare to see gene mutations in people younger than 40, gene mutations are increasingly observed in people as they age. About 10% of people older than 65 showed gene mutations and about 20% of people older than 90 showed gene mutations.

This data suggests that the increase of gene mutations is the result of long term exposure to toxic substances throughout the lifetime, and these gene mutations subsequently result in hematologic cancers such as leukemia and lymphoma. Pre-cancer cells wait silently in the blood of many older people and their increased presence heightens the risk of cancer. Usually, several gene mutations need to occur before a cell turns abnormal and transforms into a cancerous cell. Having just one mutation will not necessarily lead to the development of blood cancer, but this will increase the risk of cancer by more than 10 times as well as the risk of heart attack or stroke, which can cause a reduction of one's lifespan.

Interestingly, two independent study teams have found that there are three gene mutations that can lead to the development of blood cancer. One of the gene mutations can trigger blood cancer within one year in 1% of blood cancer patients and within 12 years in 10% of blood cancer patients. The studies also found that people with one of the blood-gene mutations had more than twice the risk of heart attack and stroke.

These results have important implications for further research that may reveal the origins of some blood cancers.

References

1. Dr. Benjamin Ebert of Brigham and Women's Hospital in Boston.
2. Dr. Janis Abkowitz, Blood Diseases Chief at the University of Washington in Seattle and past President of the American Society of Hematology, *New England Journal of Medicine*, November 26, 2014.

Consumption of Soybean Protein for Breast Cancer Patients

There has been some discussion about the pros and cons of soy protein consumption for breast cancer patients.

Some reports have suggested that soy may interfere with anti-cancer drugs while others have suggested that isoflavones in soy mimic estrogen which can fuel some breast cancers. A study by the National Cancer Institute (NCI) in 2014 reported that soybean proteins can promote the activity of genes related to the growth of breast cancer.

However, several studies also showed that women who eat a good amount of soy everyday were less likely to experience recurrence or die of breast cancer than women who consumed less soy.

A recent study[1] by Dr. Fang F. Zhang *et al.* from the Friedman School of Nutrition Science and Policy at Tufts University reported that soy consumption may not be that harmful for women with breast cancer after all, and that soy-based foods may even provide protective benefits. Dr. Zhang *et al.* reported in the journal *Cancer* that, over a study period of nine years, breast cancer patients who ate more soy did not have a higher risk of dying compared to women who consumed less. Among patients with a particular type of breast cancer, eating soy also appeared to lower the risk of dying from any cause during that observation period.

The data of more than 6,200 women diagnosed with different types of breast cancer was analyzed in Dr. Zhang's study. This pool of breast cancer patients included patients who were driven by estrogen as well as those who were not, and the patients reported on their diet. The type of treatments the women received were analyzed to see if their soy ingestion affected their response.

The data showed that women who ate more soy (a half to one serving a week) were 21% less likely to die of any cause than women who ate less soy over the nine years observation period.

A sub-analysis of the data according to the type of breast cancer showed that breast cancer patients with estrogen- and progesterone-negative cancers that were not driven by hormones accounted for most of the decline in mortality rate. But even women who had estrogen- and progesterone-positive cancers appeared not to be harmed by soy. There was also no increase in mortality for patients who were taking anti-estrogen drugs to treat the cancer. This indicates that the soy protein did not make the anti-estrogen drug treatment ineffective.

While more studies are needed to confirm these findings, women with breast cancer do not have to avoid soy because there is no solid evidence demonstrating the harmfulness of soy toward breast cancer patients.

Reference

1. Dr. Zhang, Friedman School of Nutrition Science and Policy at Tufts University, Soy Food Consumption Linked to Prolonged Survival in Some Breast Cancer Patients, Cancer Online, March 2017.

Risk of Stroke in Cancer Patients

Cancer patients face a much higher risk of stroke compared to cancer-free senior individuals, independent of other risk factors like high blood pressure and diabetes. The risk of stroke was the highest in cancer patients when the intensity of chemotherapy, radiation, and other treatments was highest, especially during the first three months after cancer diagnosis.[1]

The study did not examine why the risk of stroke should be higher in cancer patients, but cancer and its treatments seem to affect blood vessels and the blood clotting system, causing the blood to be thicken.[1] Hence, cancer patients should be vigilant and immediately call for medical help when they experience any signs and symptoms of stroke.

Reference

1. Association between incident cancer and subsequent stroke, *Ann Neurol* 2015;**77**(2):291–300.

Rotating Night Shift Workers Face Higher Risk of Cancer and Heart Disease

Although it is difficult to prove that night shift work causes disease, an article reported that night shift work may have detrimental impact on health. People who work at least three nights per month are classified as doing rotating night shift work.

The study included about 75,000 female registered nurses in the US. The research team followed the women for 22 years from 1988 to 2010 and reviewed their weight, diet, and lifestyle. When 14,181 women had died by 2010, the study collected the dates and causes of death.

The following are the key points from the report[1]:

- There was 11% higher risk of death in women who did rotating night shift work for more than five years regardless of the specific cause of death compared to women who did not.
- Heart disease-related mortality was 19% higher in women who did rotating night shift work for 6 to 14 years compared than women who did not.
- Women who did rotating night shifts for more than 15 years had a 23% higher mortality rate than women who did not.
- Women who worked on rotating night shifts for more than 15 years had a 25% higher mortality rate due to the lung cancer compared to women who did not.

In addition, women who worked on rotating night shifts for longer periods were usually older (mean age 66), heavier, more likely to smoke, and less likely to take postmenopausal hormones or multivitamins. Compared to women who do not do rotating night shift work, they tend to drink more alcohol and eat less cereal or fiber daily, and they were also more likely to have diabetes, high blood pressure, and high cholesterol.[1]

Reference

1. Dr. Eva Schernhammer of Harvard Medical School; *American Journal of Preventive Medicine*, March 2014.

Natural Food and Alternative Therapies

Natural food showing anti-angiogenesis effects

Blood vessels are normally generated (angiogenesis) when the body is recovering from physical injury or when a woman becomes pregnant and the placenta is created. However, abnormal generation of blood vessels will encourage the growth of cancer cells. Cancer cells generate micro-blood vessels to obtain nutrients for survival and growth. If the generation of micro-blood vessels by cancer cells is blocked, the growth of cancer cells will be stopped.

Sometimes, we observe cancer patients surviving for many years by eating natural food and without experiencing adverse effects. It is difficult to know exactly what specific biochemical reactions occur in the body when natural food is consumed, but there should be certain mechanisms in natural food that work against cancer cells.

Several research papers[1-3] have described some natural foods that show an anti-angiogenesis effect or the inhibition of micro-blood vessels formation. Some examples are red wine, grapes (resveratrol), tea (polyphenols), eggplant (nasunin), and carrots and vegetables (carotenoids). Several types of functional foods containing anti-angiogenic ingredients are available in the market.[4]

References

1. E. Brakenhielm. (2001) *FASEB*.
2. Y. Cao. (2002) *Journal of Nutritional Biochemistry*.
3. K. Matsubara. (2005) *ACS*.
4. S. Kuhnen. (2009) *Journal of Functional Foods*.

AHCC mushroom extracts — natural anti-cancer agent

HPV is a cause of infection to the genitalia (e.g., vulva, vagina, penis, and anus), and HPV infection is the leading cause of cervical cancer. In October 2014, Dr. Judith A. Smith reported at the 11th International Conference of the Society for Integrative Oncology that a mushroom extract known as active hexose correlated compound (AHCC) is effective in eradicating HPV infection.[1]

The research team conducted a clinical study on 10 subjects with HPV infection. The subjects were treated with 3 g of AHCC for six months. The results of the study showed that HPV infection had disappeared in 6 subjects. The other four subjects continued being treated with AHCC as the study report said that the effect of AHCC was slow and could only show its effectiveness after at least 6 months of continuous treatment.

The research team also showed the efficacy of AHCC by studying its mechanism of action with animal models. AHCC boosted the immune system by activating interferon (interferon)-α, β, and γ in the body, thereby eradicating HPV 16 and HPV 18.

A Phase 2 clinical trial was planned based on the positive results of the AHCC treatment. In addition, the team was planning another study using AHCC to remove warts formed by HPV in the genitalia mucous membranes and the anus.

Reference

1. Judith A. Smith, Pharm D, Department of Obstetrics, Gynaecology and Reproductive Sciences at the University of Texas Health Sciences Center at Houston Medical School; Abstract 138 presented October 26, 2014 at the 11th International Conference of the Society for Integrative Oncology.

Effects of Herbal Medicine and Nutritional Supplements on Cancer Patients under Chemotherapy

Wise use of herbal medicine and nutritional supplements

Chemical interactions may occur between anti-cancer drugs and herbal medicine or certain nutritional supplements, which may lead to harmful adverse effects on cancer patients. In one survey, 400 American oncology doctors stated that they do not discuss about herbal medicine or nutritional supplements with their patients. The main reason for not having such discussions is due to their lack of knowledge about herbal medicine and nutritional supplements.

Many cancer patients take functional foods, natural foods, and herbal medicine to improve their health condition as well as to fight cancer. Although herbal medicine and nutritional supplements are perceived as natural food, some active ingredients in herbal medicine or nutritional supplements can interact with anti-cancer drugs, leading to adverse effects. Some supplements were found to induce skin irritation in cancer patients receiving radiation therapy. Herbal medicine or supplements may also interfere with absorption and metabolism of anti-cancer drugs in the body.[1]

One study identified herbs such as St. John's wort, ginseng, and green tea in herbal medicine which can interact with chemotherapy drugs and cause dangerous chemical reactions in the body.[1]

Patients undergoing chemotherapy are advised not to take herbal medicines or functional food supplements in order to avoid adverse effects from drug interactions. If patients want to take herbal medicine or functional foods to boost their health condition or immune system, it is better to do so only after chemotherapy and radiation therapy is completed.

Reference

1. Richard Lee, MD, Assistant Professor, Department of General Oncology, Division of Cancer Medicine, Medical Director, Integrative Medicine Program, University of Texas MD Anderson Cancer Center, Houston, *Journal of Clinical Oncology*, January 5, 2015. The Contents discussed by Dr. Patricia Ganz, Medical Oncologist.

Alternative Medicine versus Conventional Cancer Therapies

To understand the effects of alternative medicine on cancer treatment, a research team reviewed the National Cancer Database from 2004 to 2013 with a focus on four common cancers: breast, lung, colorectal, and prostate.

Compared to the conventional treatment patient group, the alternative medicine patient group was younger, more likely to have breast or lung cancer, better educated, more affluent, and more likely to have Stage II or III disease, and they also had lower comorbidity scores. These comparisons suggest that the patients who opted for alternative medicine were in a relatively better condition or situation, and thus could potentially be cured.[1]

However, the patients who chose alternative medicine as the only treatment for potentially curable cancers had significantly worse survival rates when compared with similar patients who received conventional treatments such as chemotherapy, surgery, radiotherapy, and hormonal therapy.[1]

Overall, the 5-year survival rate for the alternative medicine group was 54.7% versus the conventional treatment group's 78.3%.

The 5-year survival rates for each type of cancer in terms of alternative medicines versus conventional treatment are as follows[1]:

- Breast cancer: 58.1% versus 86.6%;
- Lung cancer: 19.9% versus 41.3%;
- Colorectal cancer: 32.7% versus 79.4%; and
- Prostate cancer: 86.2% versus 91.5% (not significantly different).

In conclusion, cancer patients who initially chose treatment with alternative medicines without conventional treatments were more likely to die earlier.

Reference

1. Johnson SB, *et al.* (2018) Use of alternative medicine for cancer and its impact on survival. *J Nat Cancer Inst* **110**:121–124.

Chapter 14

The Right for Patients to Opt for Death

Should terminal-stage cancer patients who are suffering from constant intolerable pain be given the right to choose death?

In this book, we have discussed two important concerns for terminal cancer patients. The first is to protect the patient's dignity and decency from excess medical treatment. Second, adequate hospice care and services should be provided for patients so that they can spend the last part of their life as comfortably as possible.

In addition to the previous discussion on the excessive medical treatment and hospice services, we will now discuss a kind of advanced and controversial concept of euthanasia or assisted suicide. The debate over whether patients have the right to determine their own death by opting for physician-assisted euthanasia has been ongoing for many years in many states and countries.

By 2015, five European countries (Netherlands, Belgium, Luxembourg, Switzerland, and France) have allowed certain patients to opt for physician-assisted euthanasia. Oregon's right-to-die law, also known as Death with Dignity, was started in 1997. By 2015, certain patients in Washington, Montana, New Mexico, Vermont, and California may opt for physician-assisted euthanasia. In 2015, California passed a bill to do up a legislation for physician-assisted euthanasia.

Discussions on such legislations are actively going on in more countries around the world. In the US, New Jersey, New York, and Connecticut are actively working on the bill.[1] However, the pros and cons of this legislation are very controversial.

The bill for euthanasia is only for terminal-stage patients with irreversible disease accompanied with chronic pain. These patients can be allowed to terminate their lives with support from physicians.

Janet Colbert has been working as a nurse at a cancer center in New Jersey for more than 20 years. Over the course of her work, Janet said that she had been asked by several terminal-stage cancer patients to help end their lives.

Now at 69 years of age, Janet has liver cancer and wishes to terminate her life as she does not want to go through the long process of death accompanied by excruciating pain in the body. In other words, she wishes to exercise the right to choose a peaceful death using assisted suicide rather than prolong life meaninglessly.

However, the outcome of the discussions over the legislation is inconclusive as there are strong objections from several organizations, including the Roman Catholic Church, American Medical Association, and some groups representing people with disabilities.

Dissenting organizations argue that the concept of legislation allowing for assisted suicide is very dangerous and morally wrong in the eyes of the law.

The key points of the dissenters' arguments are:

- Allowing terminally ill patients to end their lives implies that something is undignified about natural death.

- Assisted suicide can be acceptable to some people, but not acceptable to others. This will present a contradictory message to people.
- The Catholic Church is suggests that there are alternatives to assisted suicide, such as hospice and palliative care for terminally ill patients.
- The Bill would give people the legal authority to end their life earlier than their actual life expectancy.
- The value of life in people with disabilities will be undermined.

On the other hand, the supporters' arguments are:

- It is not right to equate committing suicide with the decision made by terminally ill patients to end their lives with the help of physicians.
- If terminally ill patients are not suffering from prolonged excruciating pain, they will choose to live rather than die.

New Jersey Democratic Assemblyman, John Burzichelli, said a careful reading of the key points of the legislated Bill will show that the arguments of dissenters are groundless.

Let's take look at the core items of the proposed legislation:

- People who are chronically ill or with disabilities should not be defined as terminally ill. There are clear descriptions in the Bill about terminal disease.
- An attending physician and a consulting physician must determine that the patient who wishes to have assisted

suicide is indeed suffering from a terminal disease and will die within six months.

- The patient must make one written and oral request first, followed by a second oral request at least 15 days later.
- Two witnesses, including one non-relative, would need to be present to witness the signing of the written request.
- Patients would administer the medication to themselves.

While legislators are trying to push the Bill ahead, it looks like governors in the region are not in favor of the idea.

Reference

1. Joseph De Avila, Feb. 16, 2015. Bills Would Let Doctors Help Terminally Ill Patients End Their Lives; Measures in New Jersey, New York and Connecticut Legislatures.

Closing: The War Against Cancer

Since President Nixon declared war on cancer in 1971 to the end of 2014, more than US$90 billion has been invested on cancer research in the US. Thanks to the great support for the last several decades, incredibly advanced technologies for the diagnosis and treatment of cancer have been developed and made available for cancer patients around the world.

Owing to the advances in medical technology, the overall survival time after the diagnosis of cancer has been extended from a few weeks or months in the past to several years now. Although treatment results differ from patient to patient depending on the types of cancer and conditions they have, we can even see some cancer patients getting completely cured these days.

As innovative drugs are continuously emerging, drugs in the future should be able to provide cancer patients with even better efficacy, leading to longer survival periods and having less toxicities. Along with the superior efficacy of advanced cancer drugs, if cancer patients diligently work and take advantage of rehabilitation programs with a strong emphasis on exercise, nutrition, and symptom control (side effect management), they would still be able to live a long and good quality life.

Scientific research is continuing to develop new innovative drugs to exceed the current best class of drugs in terms of efficacy and toxicity. Some examples include innovative technologies using re-engineered viruses, genetically modified bacteria, target drugs combined with chemotherapy drugs, uniquely designed CART-T cell immunotherapy, and immunotherapy drugs such as programmed cell death protein 1 (PD-1)/programmed cell death ligand 1 (PD-L1) inhibitors.

In addition, the availability of gigantic pools of accumulated clinical data and personal genetic information will be another important complement to the treatment of various types of cancers.

Just like measles and smallpox which were conquered by specific vaccines developed several decades ago, cancer should also be conquered eventually by future innovative therapies. Cancer will then be classified as a curable disease someday in the future.

An Order

The basic elements of life — DNA and its genetic information — are programmed to sustain life and reproduce a new life, thereby enabling the life to continue from generation to generation. The life cycles of birth, aging, illness, and death will carry on according to the biological program that has already been pre-set by our genetic information.

The cells in our body are diligently doing their job to sustain the integrity of the whole body. Cells in the body are dying at certain time points and being replaced by new cells throughout the whole life cycle.

When cells lose their ability to perform their functions due to aging or damage caused by other factors, the old or damaged cells will negatively impact or burden neighboring cells or tissues, resulting in the weakening of whole tissues or organs. When this situation occurs, the body sends out an order, signaling the non-functioning cells to commit suicide and get dismantled. By removing the damaged old cells and replacing them with newborn cells, the body keeps the entire organ healthy and strong.

If we link the phenomena of recycling of old cells with newborn cells in the body to the onset of cancer in human beings, the onset of cancer would be a kind of genetically programmed order to effectively sustain human beings, by replacing old generation of people with a new healthy generation.

Owing to the wonderful advances in science and technology, the current life expectancy of humans is almost doubled compared to the average life expectancy at the time of World War I, which was only around a century ago. However, despite the incredible advances in science and technology today, the maximum lifespan of a human hardly goes beyond 115 years.

The lifespan has been set by the biological program in each individual. As the needle of the clock moves forward every second, all of us are taking one more step towards death. This means while we are living every day, we are also dying at the same time. My clock will also stop some day in the future.

Death is sometimes referred to as a new start. However, this new start would not be for myself but it would be for the next generation instead. When we are dying, it would be a great fortune if we can encounter and hold to a new light at the end of the tunnel which bring us to the start of a new journey. Now, the mission left for us is to complete our remaining journey as happy as possible, and then to move through the last exit with dignity.

Index

www.ingramcontent.com/pod-product-compliance
Lightning Source LLC
Chambersburg PA
CBHW061251220326
41599CB00028B/5604